"This book is a must for anyone who is breathing the air, eating the food, and drinking the water on this incredibly polluted planet. For those who are no longer able to breathe, eat and drink, this book is unfortunately too late. Although we can not seem to stop the merciless polluters, or activate the slow-to-respond governments at this point in time, this book offers a powerful way for us to protect ourselves from the all-encompassing pollution, that is poisoning our enzyme systems—so that we can not heal or repair, depleting brain function in everyone, contributing mightily to autism, depleting our ATP energy production systems, accelerating the aging process, and ultimately our physical, emotional, mental, and spiritual joy in life. Chelation is not only a reasonable self-defense or nice prevention idea; it is a must for the survival of our endangered human species."

—Gabriel Cousens, M.D., M.D.(h), Diplomat in Ayurveda, American Board of Holistic Medicine and author of *There Is A Cure For Diabetes* and *Conscious Eating*

Dr. Garry Gordon, you have been a personal inspiration to many physicians and patients worldwide in the field of Integrative Medicine. I personally follow many of your teachings myself and am looking forward to a longer and healthier life directly because I take your advice and use your supplements on a daily basis. I've had the privelege of working with you on the AZ Homeopathic Board, and furthering the cause of our style of medicine up against some over-reaching odds—and we have succeeded. You are one of my personal Medical Heroes!

— Bruce H. Shelton M.D., M.D.(h) DiHom FBIH
Homeopathic Family Physician (www.drbruceshelton.com)

Are you concerned about the heavy metal toxicity that you are guaranteed to have simply by living on polluted planet Earth? Do you have any chronic degenerative illnesses? Have you been misled by your conventional doctor about chelation therapy? Has even your alternative doctor discouraged the use and effectiveness of oral chelation therapy? Are you ready for an easy to read and understand treatise on perhaps the simplest thing you can do to enhance your health and protect against degenerative disease (other than a pristine diet)? Are you interested in an inexpensive yet effective alternative to intravenous treatments for heavy metal toxicity? If you have answered yes to any of these questions, this book is indispensible. The authors dramatically and accurately (with references) educate you on a totally neglected (by conventional medicine) cause of disease affecting 100% of the earth's inhabitants to one extent or another. Even better, they provide information on affordable remedies.

There are only three major causes of disease: malnutrition, stress and toxins. This book does a better job at addressing a most serious cause of universal toxicity than any publication in the field. This is a must read book for lay people and health professionals alike who have any interest in preventing disease and treating the cause, not the symptoms.

—Robert Jay Rowen, M.
internat

Newsletter and
dical Freedom"
.newsletter.com)

Detox with Oral Chelation:
Protecting Yourself from Lead, Mercury, & Other Environmental Toxins

David Jay Brown & Garry Gordon, M.D.

Illustrations by Sara Huntley

DETOX WITH ORAL CHELATION
David Jay Brown & Garry Gordon, M.D.

Published by:

SmartPublications™

PO Box 4667
Petaluma, CA 94955
www.smart-publications.com

**Published in the United States of America
First Edition, 2009**

Library of Congress Control Number: 2008929521

ISBN: 1-890572-20-9   978-1-890572-20-4

Warning—Disclaimer

TABLE OF CONTENTS

For

Steven Ray Brown, a.k.a. Sammie Rose

~David

For

Alexandra Van Cleve—Who has inspired me to devote my life to educating others about the dangers of pollution and the dramatically improved Health and Longevity Oral Chelation provides.

Today's rapidly increasing levels of pollution has made continuous Oral Chelation-based Detox essential for anyone hoping to reach their maximum intended useful lifespan, while enjoying optimal health.

The clear evidence is in this book—we all need to "get the lead out"!

~Garry

Acknowledgments

This book was largely the brainchild of Dr. Garry Gordon. I enthusiastically agreed to coauthoring this book with Dr. Gordon after interviewing him for my book *Mavericks of Medicine*, and then trying chelation therapy myself with spectacular results.

Dr. Gordon would like to thank Linus Pauling and Robert C. Atkins.

I would like to extend extra special thanks to Sara Huntley for the wonderful illustrations that she did for this book.

I would also like to express my appreciation to the following individuals for their valuable help: Carolyn Mary Kleefeld, John Morgenthaler, Ron Williams, Dr. Jerry Schlesser, Gerhard N. Schrauzer, Durk Pearson, Nancy Guyon, Sandra Litkenhaus, Chris Higgins, Cynthia Deyoung, Danell Loy, Randy Baker, Richard Goldberg, Louise Reitman, Arleen Margulis, Jenna Sunde, Erin Dellinger, Jessi Daichman, Amy Barnes Excolere, Sherry Hall, Serena Watman, Amanda Rose Loveland, Jesse Ray Houts, Steven Ray Brown, Joe & Suzie Wouk, Valerie Leveroni Corral, David Wayne Dunn, Linda Parker, Patricia Holt, Robin Rae & Brummbaer, B'anna Federico, Rick Doblin, Sarah Hufford, Jag Davies, Valerie Mojeiko, Joshua Sonstroem, Anna Damoth, Sandy Oppenheim, Lorey Capelli, Dana Peleg, Mimi Hill, Sherri Paris, Deed DeBruno, Bethan Carter, Al Brown, Cheryle and Gene Goldstein, Sammie and Tudie, Bernadette Wilson, Nick Herbert, Erin Jarvis, Jody Lombardo, Erica Ansberry, Taylor Burns, Maria Ramirez, Robert Forte, and Paula Rae Mellard.

I would also like to express my sincere gratitude to the people that I interviewed for their valuable time and generous help with this project.

INTRODUCTION

An abundance of compelling scientific evidence suggests that EDTA chelation therapy can dramatically enhance many people's health and performance. EDTA chelation therapy has been shown to help prevent arteriosclerosis[1] and cancer[2], improve blood circulation[3], lower blood pressure[4], reduce harmful clotting mechanisms[5], and remove lead and other toxic heavy metals from the body.[6]

Some of the other reported benefits from EDTA chelation therapy include better skin texture and skin tone, improvements with arthritis, and better vision and hearing. It has also been shown to improve conditions with renal function and macular degeneration[7], and to reduce blood pressure and cholesterol levels.[8] Although EDTA chelation therapy has been shown to reduce calcium accumulation in the blood vessels, it is actually used as a treatment for osteoporosis because it has been shown to stimulate bone growth and to make bones stronger.[9]

EDTA chelation therapy has been reported to dramatically improve physical energy levels, which a number of researchers suspect is due to mitochondrial stimulation, as it is known that lead interferes with mitochondrial function[10] and chelation therapy helps to remove lead from the body. EDTA chelation therapy is also known to have antiviral and antioxidant activity.[11] Perhaps most importantly, because it increases circulation to the brain, EDTA chelation therapy may also help to improve cognitive function and memory.[12] Others have reported that using EDTA can have an antidepressant effect. In other words, in addition to making us stronger and healthier, EDTA chelation therapy may actually help to make us smarter and happier.

What is EDTA Chelation Therapy?

Since 1956 over a million people have been treated with EDTA chelation therapy, yet most people don't even know that this unusually safe, relatively inexpensive, and remarkably effective therapy exists, and far too many doctors are unfamiliar with the scientific studies that demonstrate its myriad of benefits.

The word "chelation" comes from the Greek word, *chele*, meaning "claw" or the grabbing appendage of a crab or lobster. Chelation is a chemical process in which a metal or mineral—such as lead, mercury, or calcium—is bonded to another substance. This is a natural process that goes on continually in our bodies. For example, the transportation and migration of zinc and iron in and out of cells are achieved by a chelating process, and the iron in hemoglobin is a chelated metal.

A chelate is a chemical compound in which the central atom is attached to neighboring atoms by at least two bonds in such a way as to form a ring structure. This central atom is usually a metal ion, and during the process of chelation it reacts with other metals and minerals in the body and binds with them. Chelation therapy generally employs the weak acid EDTA, although we will be discussing some other important chelators in this book, such as garlic, vitamin C, and malic acid.

EDTA (ethylenediaminetetraacetic acid) is a synthetic amino acid, which is essentially composed of four molecules of vinegar, and is often used as a food preservative. It was first synthesized in Germany in 1935, and then patented in the U.S. in 1941. In chelation therapy EDTA is administered either orally or intravenously (I.V.) in a doctor's office. The difference between these two methods of administration, and an assessment of their relative benefits, will be discussed later in the book.

Initially, EDTA chelation was used as a way for workers in early battery factories, or for those who painted ships with lead-based paints, to remove lead or other toxic heavy metals from their body after they had been exposed to high levels because of their jobs. To this day, this is the one area that conventional medicine accepts chelation as a form of treatment—heavy metal poisoning, especially lead poisoning. EDTA is incredibly effective at removing lead and other dangerous heavy metals from the body. However, not long after EDTA first came into use, it was soon reported that people who received chelation treatments for lead poisoning were also experiencing cardiovascular benefits— such as a reduction in symptoms of heart disease—and other health improvements.

Scientific Research on EDTA

The scientific evidence supporting the benefits of EDTA chelation therapy is quite substantial. Early research conducted at the Providence Hospital in Detroit, Michigan in 1955 found that EDTA dissolves "metastatic calcium"—i.e., unwanted calcium deposits.[13] In the first systematic study of EDTA—which was published a year later—twenty patients with confirmed heart disease were given a series of thirty intravenous EDTA treatments. Nineteen of the patients experienced improvement, as measured by an increase in physical activity.[14] Then, in 1960, another study found that three months of EDTA treatments caused a decrease in the severity and frequency of anginal episodes, increased work capacity, improved electrocardiogram (ECG) results, and significantly reduced the use of the anti-angina drug nitroglycerin.[15]

Since these early studies were done in the late '50s and early '60s there are now hundreds of published papers demonstrating the beneficial health effects of EDTA chelation therapy in treating a wide variety of chronic diseases. In 1993 and 1994 two large meta-analyses—where the results from many scientific studies are statistically analyzed together—evaluated the results of over 24,000 chelation treatments and eighty-eight percent of the patients demonstrated clinical improvement.[16, 17]

Because of the dramatic cardiovascular benefits that EDTA has demonstrated, for many years people believed that EDTA worked by "clawing" away calcium deposits in one's arteries and veins, or dissolving these calcified blockages like a biological version of Drano or Roto-Rooter. We now know that this assumption doesn't hold up in scientific tests. Even though EDTA dissolves metastatic calcium and improves blood circulation, studies show that it appears to have little effect on cardiovascular blockages.[18] Nonetheless, people who use EDTA continue to show improved circulation and other cardiovascular benefits. The mechanism by which these benefits occur is a bit of a mystery, although some compelling theories for the action have been proposed and will be discussed in this book.

EDTA Gets the Lead Out

My coauthor—who has been studying EDTA chelation therapy for the past twenty-five years and is considered one of the world's foremost experts on the subject—is convinced that the primary mechanism in chelation therapy for all the different benefits involves EDTA's ability to remove lead, mercury, cadmium, and other toxic heavy metals from the body. According to Dr. Gordon every person on this planet—to one degree or another—is suffering from heavy metal and pesticide poisoning. Every person alive today has around a thousand times more lead in their bones than anyone who lived prior to the Industrial Age.

Rising lead levels in the body have been linked to numerous diseases, such as the formation of cataracts in the eye[19] and an increased risk of cardiovascular disease.[20] A disturbing study at the Tulane University School of Public Health demonstrated that the average blood level of lead found among Americans is high enough to increase the likelihood of heart attack and stroke.[21] In other words, lead toxicity is ubiquitous and everyone's health is compromised to some extent as a result.

"The Earth has become so totally polluted that everybody today is walking around with high-levels of styrene, PCBs, and dioxins. They're in every human being we test today, as well as is lead, mercury, and cadmium. There is simply no escape from the particulate matter. We have poisoned our nest," Dr. Gordon told me.

Because lead and zinc are so closely related to each other chemically, when we raise the levels of lead in our body we are actually plugging lead into key enzyme functions that normally zinc would have fulfilled. According to Dr. Gordon, this is severely compromising many biological functions, and by using EDTA chelation therapy we restore many of these vital functions to their original capacity.

For example, it is suspected that EDTA has a stimulating effect on the mitochondria in our cells, as it is known that lead interferes with mitochondrial activity.[22] Mitochondria are structures within cells that produce energy—in the form of the molecule ATP (adenosine triphosphate)—by respiratory metabolism, and many researchers believe that the loss of mitochondrial function is one of the primary causes of aging. Because zinc is so important for intracellular processes, removing the lead and replacing it with zinc may be one of the keys to slowing down the aging process.

EDTA has also been shown to optimize nitric oxide production.[23] Nitric oxide helps to protect the heart and dilate the arteries, among many other vital functions in the body. Dr. Gordon believes that having lead plugged into those key enzymes functions in our body that zinc normally would have fulfilled inhibits nitric oxide synthesis. This is because some of those enzymes are nitric oxide syntheses, the key enzymes that are responsible for this job of making nitric oxide out of the arginine and related amino acids that we get in our diet.

Why Don't More Physicians Practice EDTA Chelation Therapy?

Although a review of the scientific literature supports the assertion that EDTA chelation therapy can have numerous beneficial effects, the official position from the American Heart Association (AHA) on chelation therapy is that "there is no scientific evidence that demonstrates any benefit from this form of therapy in the treatment of arteriosclerotic heart disease."

Although the AHA recognizes chelation therapy as a treatment for heavy metal poisoning, and EDTA chelation therapy is the standard FDA treatment for heavy metal poisoning, neither the American Medical Association or the FDA acknowledge it as a treatment for heart disease or for many of its other demonstrated health benefits. Organizations like the American Heart Association and the American Medical Association, which say that EDTA chelation is ineffective for treating vascular disease usually quote several Danish and New Zealand studies to support their position.

However, what these titanic organizations fail to mention is that the Danish studies were actually criticized by the Danish Committee for Investigation into Scientific Dishonesty because of improper randomization and double-blinding, as well as premature breaking of the blinding code.[24] This amounted to a deliberate bias. When the results of the New Zealand study were examined by two independent statisticians, it was concluded that the trial actually supported the efficacy of EDTA.[25]

However, as a result of these official denouncements of chelation therapy, many people simply dismiss it as though it were some kind of New Age quackery, and those who support chelation therapy tend to support the notion that this misinformation about chelation therapy was deliberately spread by these official organizations because the patent on EDTA ran out long ago and the pharmaceutical companies can no longer profit from it.

Cardiovascular surgery is an enormously profitable enterprise and the medical community would lose a substantial portion of its profits if an inexpensive and equally effective treatment were to be offered as an alternative. Coronary artery bypass surgery alone is an 18.4 billion dollar a year industry. Many people believe that this is the primary reason why—despite the scientific evidence supporting its many dramatic health benefits—EDTA chelation therapy is not more widely practiced.[26] Support for this point of view comes from a study where sixty-five patients on a waiting list for coronary artery bypass surgery were treated with EDTA chelation therapy and the symptoms in eighty-nine percent improved so much that they were able to cancel their surgery.[27] The numerous scientific studies that support the many benefits of EDTA chelation therapy will be discussed in this book.

Currently the National Institutes of Health (NIH) has a five year study underway, involving 2,372 participants. This is the first large scale study looking at whether EDTA chelation therapy is "safe and effective for people with coronary heart disease," and although twenty-nine million dollars is being spent on the study some chelation-practicing physicians have strong criticisms of this work, which will also be discussed in this book.

When I asked Dr. Gordon why he thought oral EDTA chelation therapy isn't recommended by more physicians he said, "I think this is because the standard policy of doctors is to be down on what they're not up on...the scientific literature in this country is entirely controlled. The net result is that if you have a real breakthrough, something that's really going to cure cancer or heart disease, it's not going to be in the *New England Journal of Medicine* or *The Lancet* because of the game that is played in this world. We've known from the beginning that this was too big a revolution. If every doctor did what I'm promoting there would be no huge hospitals."

Why Do So Many People Believe in EDTA Chelation Therapy?

Many people hear about EDTA chelation by word of mouth from people who experienced benefits from it themselves. In writing this book, I conducted a series of interviews with Dr. Gordon and a number of other chelation specialists, as well as some of the patients who have experienced dramatic improvements with chelation therapy. Excerpts from these interviews will be included throughout the book in order to give a sense of how chelation therapy can really affect people's lives.

The late Linus Pauling—the only person ever to have received two full, unshared Nobel Prizes—strongly supported chelation therapy while he was alive. In fact, Dr. Pauling wrote the forward to *A Textbook on EDTA Chelation Therapy* by Elmer Cranton, M.D. In his forward Dr. Pauling states, "EDTA chelation therapy makes good sense to me as a chemist and medical researcher. It has a rational scientific basis, and the evidence for clinical benefit seems to be quite strong...The scientific evidence indicates that a course of EDTA chelation therapy might eliminate the need for bypass surgery. Chelation has an equally valid rationale for use as a preventive treatment. Past harassment of chelating physicians by government agencies and conservative medical societies seems to stem largely from ignorance of the scientific literature and from professional bias."

I enthusiastically agreed to writing this book with Dr. Gordon after interviewing him for my book *Mavericks of Medicine* and then trying EDTA chelation therapy myself. The very first day I tried oral EDTA I was astonished by the effects and I've been using it regularly ever since. Several hours after taking EDTA orally for the first time I experienced significantly more energy and was able to think more clearly. Most impressively, it completely lifted me out of a mild depression that I had been experiencing. I've spoken with many other people who have experienced similar effects.

How Safe is EDTA Chelation Therapy?

EDTA has an unparalleled history of over forty years of safe use. It has been shown to be hundreds of times safer than aspirin. The most important thing to know about EDTA safety is that you need to take a good quality multi-mineral supplement when you are on chelation therapy because it could potentially remove essential minerals. EDTA binds to the metals and minerals in your bloodstream so it's important to replace these essential nutrients when you're on a chelation therapy program.

However, it's important to note that in some instances EDTA actually enhances the uptake of various trace minerals. In fact, the World Health Organization and advisors to the National Academy of Science recommend that EDTA be added to the diet of children in poor countries to enhance mineral absorption, particularly of iron and zinc.

Many years ago there were some reports of renal (kidney) damage and other adverse effects which resulted from excessive doses of EDTA, infused too rapidly (more than 50 mg/Kg/day or infused more rapidly than 16.6 mg/min), especially in the presence of a preexisting kidney disease. However, when administered with the new protocol no serious side effects have been reported, yet some people still erroneously believe that EDTA can cause kidney damage. Ironically, studies done in 2003 and 2007 by Ja-Liang Lin and colleagues provides evidence that EDTA chelation therapy may actually improve renal function in people with renal disease whose kidneys have been exposed to environmental lead.[28],[29]

According to Dr. Gordon, EDTA chelation therapy has an extremely low risk of side-effects—less than one in ten thousand people. "EDTA is never broken down in the body. It goes in and comes out as EDTA, so it's hard for it to do a lot of mischief," Dr. Gordon said. When administered by a proper physician, and carried out according to accepted protocols, mortality rates for EDTA chelation therapy approach zero percent.

Following the guidelines of the American College of Advancement in Medicine (ACAM), more than a million patients have received over twenty million treatments without a single fatality attributed to EDTA.

This claim can not even be made for aspirin, let alone any surgical procedure.

EDTA Provides Extreme Detoxification

Until we develop the nanotechnological expertise to detoxify our bodies with sub cellular robots and molecular-sized cleaning vessels, EDTA chelation therapy appears to be the safest and most effective way to cleanse our bodies of pervasive heavy metal toxins and remove age-accelerating calcium deposits from our cardiovascular systems. It also appears to be the safest and most effective way to help thin our blood and prevent the formation of blood clots, lower blood pressure and cholesterol levels, and neutralize dangerous free radicals.

The accumulating scientific evidence suggests that this mighty amino acid offers a whole range of truly remarkable health benefits, and it seems prudent to suggest that everyone on this planet should consider taking EDTA. According to Dr. Gordon, "Every human being today would live longer, be more intelligent, have a higher level of health, and respond better to any medicine, drug, or surgery, if they chose to follow an EDTA chelation therapy program."

In a day and age where astonishing new advances in medicine are made almost daily, and our vision of the future of medicine borders on the miraculous, this overlooked, inexpensive, and often misunderstood form of therapy offers us the hope that we can all live longer, healthier, and happier lives right now. In the pages that follow we will explore these many benefits of EDTA chelation therapy and provide you with enough knowledge to start your own program today.

Chapter 1

A BRIEF HISTORY OF EDTA CHELATION THERAPY

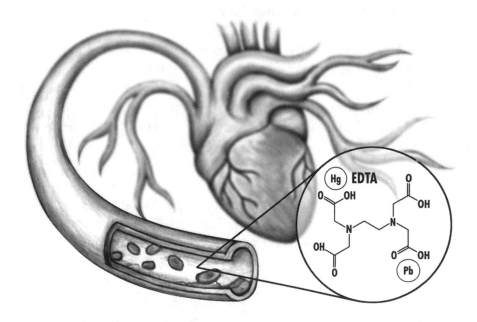

At the time of this writing, typing the word "chelation" into Amazon. com's search engine brings up eighty-nine book titles, with publication dates ranging from 1960 to the present. With so much already written about chelation therapy, why write yet another book? There are several important reasons.

First of all, the fact that there has been considerable and consistent interest in chelation therapy over the years—despite the lack of endorsement from conventional medical authorities—reflects that something important is going on. A compelling argument can be made for the notion that no medical treatment is really practiced for very long, and doesn't gain wide acceptance, if there isn't at least some truth behind its claims. For example, Western medicine's initial rejection of acupuncture and Chinese medicine—which had been practiced in the East with great success for hundreds of years—changed to reluctant acceptance once scientific studies began validating its effectiveness and mechanisms of action were discovered.

Over a thousand physicians are currently using EDTA chelation therapy in their practice in the United States and hundreds of thousands of patients have been treated with chelation therapy over the years. Despite persecution, ridicule, and even the risk of losing one's medical license, these courageous physicians have demonstrated the remarkable safety and efficiency of EDTA chelation therapy.

Although hundreds of scientific studies have demonstrated that a wide range of health benefits can be brought about through chelation therapy, and hundreds of thousands of people have experienced these benefits, most physicians remain completely unaware of this. Even worse, because the medical establishment refuses to acknowledge the benefits of chelation therapy, many doctors and much of the public have come to think that it is largely a sham or possibly dangerous.

However, demonstrating that chelation therapy is safe and efficient is only part of what this book is about. The benefits of chelation therapy have already been amply demonstrated in hundreds of scientific studies, and in dozens of books, however the mechanism by which EDTA chelation therapy achieves these benefits has never been adequately understood—and this may be part of the reason why the conventional medical community refuses to accept chelation therapy as an effective treatment for cardiovascular disease and other ailments that it has shown efficacy in treating.

Because of the dramatic cardiovascular benefits that EDTA has demonstrated, for many years people believed that EDTA improved cardiovascular performance by dissolving away calcium blockages in one's arteries and veins, like a biological version of Liquid-Plumr®. In fact, my coauthor, Dr. Garry Gordon, was partially responsible for propagating this mistaken belief years ago because it made so much sense at the time and the evidence appeared to support it.

We now know that this assumption doesn't hold up in scientific tests. Even though studies have shown that EDTA dissolves metastatic calcium,[1] and improves blood circulation,[2] more recent research reveals that it actually has little effect on cardiovascular blockages.[3] Nonetheless, people who use EDTA continue to show significantly improved circulation, lowered blood pressure, and other cardiovascular benefits.[4] So if it's not helping to clear out the cardiovascular system of unwanted calcified junk and other obstructing mineral deposits then how is it improving circulation and cardiovascular health? A number of different theories will be explored in the chapters that follow.

It appears that the answer to this question may have been staring us in the face all along but we have simply been too blind to see it. It was known from the beginning that EDTA removes lead and other toxic heavy metals from our bodies. However, for years, no one realized that every human being on this planet is suffering from some degree of heavy metal poisoning. It now appears that, because we all live in such a densely polluted world, it is primarily through the mechanism of heavy metal removal that EDTA improves our health in so many ways.

The burning of coal and petroleum, the use of powerful pesticides in our agriculture, and other toxic chemical by-products of human civilization have dramatically changed the environment that we live in over the past century. The entire biosphere on the planet has been dramatically altered as a result of our reckless behavior. In my previous book, *Conversations on the Edge of the Apocalypse*, I tried to point out that our lack of environmental awareness and misguided actions are having environmental consequences (polluted air and water, pesticides in our food, global warming, etc.) that are threatening the very survival of our species.

In this book the central message is that we've polluted our biosphere so thoroughly that our bodies are now polluted as well, and everyone's personal health is suffering as a result. So anyone who is seriously interested in improving their health should first and foremost take action to detoxify his or her body. EDTA chelation therapy appears to be the most powerful tool that we currently have for doing this. Let's take a look at the history of EDTA.

The Origins of EDTA Chelation Therapy

The non-naturally occurring amino acid EDTA (ethylenediaminetetraacetic acid) was first synthesized in Germany in 1935 and it was patented in the U.S. in 1941. It was initially used in the 1940's as a treatment for heavy metal poisoning, and it was approved for this use in the United States by the FDA in July of 1953. EDTA was primarily used as a way for workers in early battery factories, or for those who painted ships with lead-based paints, to remove lead or other toxic heavy metals from their body after they had been exposed to high levels because of their jobs. In conventional medical practice EDTA is still widely recognized as an effective treatment for heavy metal poisoning, as well as for the emergency treatment of hypercalcemia and the control of ventricular arrhythmias associated with digitalis toxicity.

However, by the mid-50's people who received chelation treatments for lead poisoning, and their physicians, were beginning to realize that something else was going on besides a simple removal of the lead. Many of these people began experiencing dramatic cardiovascular benefits— such as a reduction in symptoms of heart disease—and other significant health improvements.

In 1956, in the *American Journal of Medical Science*, Dr. Norman Clarke —a prominent cardiologist and Chief of Research at the Providence Hospital in Detroit—reported on the improvements that he observed in twenty patients with documented angina pectoris after being treated with EDTA.[5] He reported that nineteen of the twenty patients who received EDTA had a "remarkable improvement" in symptoms. In 1960 Dr. Clarke also wrote an editorial about the benefits of chelation therapy in the *American Journal of Cardiology*,[6] and he published a paper on the treatment of occlusive vascular disease with EDTA.[7] That same year Dr. Ray Evers reported on the benefits that he observed from chelation therapy in over three thousand patients.[8] Many elated physicians now believed that they had found a miracle treatment.

Then in 1963 Drs. J.R. Kitchell and L.E. Meltzer coauthored an article reassessing their support for EDTA chelation,[9] and this article sparked the beginning of the controversy over the therapy that persists to this day. Kitchell and Meltzer, who were at Presbyterian Hospital in Philadelphia, conducted chelation research from 1959 to 1963, and initially they reported good results treating cardiovascular diseases with EDTA. Then in April of 1963, shortly after their last favorable report, Kitchell and Meltzer published a "reappraisal" article in the *American Journal of Cardiology* that questioned chelation's value.

Although Kitchell and Meltzer's results were actually quite favorable their interpretation of these results were mysteriously negative. Seventy-one percent of the patients treated experienced a subjective improvement with their symptoms, sixty-four percent had a measurable improvement with regard to exercise tolerance three months after receiving twenty chelation treatments, and forty-six percent showed improved electrocardiographic patterns. Kitchell and Meltzer concluded that chelation was not effective because some patients eventually regressed long after treatment. However, all of the patients in their study were extremely ill, and considering the poor health of the patients, some eventual worsening would be expected with any treatment—yet eighteen months following therapy, forty-six percent of the patients remained significantly improved.

Whatever motivated Kitchell and Meltzer to interpret their data so negatively, and change their position so abruptly, will remain mysterious, but some physicians, such as Drs. Elmer Cranton and James Frackelton, have speculated that the motivation behind this "reappraisal" article was the "unrealistic expectation that the emergence of bypass surgery would be a final solution."[10] Nonetheless, Kitchell and Meltzer's "reappraisal" article was largely responsible for the termination of hospital-based, academic research into chelation as a treatment for cardiovascular disease.

There were studies conducted in the late 1960's by the National Academy of Sciences/National Research Council which indicated that EDTA was considered possibly effective in the treatment of occlusive vascular disorders caused by arteriosclerosis. However, by this point, clinical experience with EDTA chelation therapy had already convinced a substantial number of physicians that it was a safe and effective treatment for atherosclerotic vascular disease, as it has been shown to consistently improve blood flow and relieve symptoms associated with the disease in greater than eighty percent of the patients treated.[11] So many physicians continued treating their patients with EDTA chelation therapy and some pushed forward with their own research.

The Legal Battles Over EDTA

In my previous book, *Mavericks of Medicine*, I pointed how courageous medical researchers who question the prevailing authority are responsible for some of medicine's greatest advances. For example, in 1847, when the Hungarian physician Ignaz Semmelweis started making the claim that puerperal fever was contagious, and that poor sanitation was responsible for spreading the illness from one new mother to another, his fellow physicians thought that he was crazy. "Wash your hands!" he shouted in the hospital maternity wards of Vienna, while the other doctors laughed.

Medical science has since vindicated Semmelweis' assertions regarding the importance of hygiene in preventing the spread of disease, however this example serves to remind us that often times the conservative and skeptical nature of medicine blinds physicians from seeing obvious and simple solutions to serious problems. This is largely due to the prevailing paradigm or belief system of a particular historical period, which determines how we interpret the results of our scientific studies. As Thomas Kuhn points out in his classic work *The Structure of Scientific Revolutions*, it often takes a full generation for a new paradigm to be fully accepted into the mainstream and many researchers take their erroneous belief systems with them to the grave. The history of EDTA chelation therapy certainly illustrates this point and it involves a landmark court decision that changed how medicine is practiced.

It is unfortunate that just as evidence was being compiled for EDTA's possible treatment of cardiovascular disease, in 1969 the patent for EDTA expired, which resulted in a loss of interest by the major pharmaceutical companies. The Kitchell and Meltzer's "reappraisal" article served to dissuade physicians from practicing chelation therapy, and it helped to prevent large institutions from conducting research with it, but the patent expiring on EDTA marked the beginning of a witch hunt on physicians who practiced EDTA chelation therapy. Nonetheless, a substantial number of physicians continued to practice chelation therapy and many patients continued to experience dramatic benefits. During the 1970's, the U.S. Government began persecuting physicians who practiced chelation therapy and threatened to take away the license from anyone who used EDTA for any other use purpose than to treat heavy metal toxicity.

This changed in 1978 when Dr. Ray Evers won an important court battle over the right to use EDTA for chelation therapy, which had far-reaching consequences into other areas of medicine. Many doctors had been persecuted by the U.S. Government for using EDTA for reasons other than those that it had been approved for, and many lost their license to practice medicine during this time. The reason for this, many people suspect, is due to the fact that EDTA chelation therapy cuts into pharmaceutical company profits. Nonetheless, many courageous physicians practiced chelation therapy anyway, in ways that were considered deviant by the FDA.

When Dr. Evers was brought to court by the U.S. Government in 1978, he challenged their allegation that he was misusing his medical expertise and he won. Dr. Evers won on the grounds that physicians are allowed to use any approved substance in any way in which they believed, due to their training, was appropriate. In other words, since EDTA was approved for lead poisoning by the FDA, the government would not be allowed to second-guess a physician's diagnosis and the doctor could use it without having to defend why he or she was using it. This legal decision had dramatic consequences on how medicine is practiced in the United States. Thanks to Dr. Evers, now any physician can prescribe any approved medication for whatever ailment he or she believes will be helped by it, without fear of losing his or her license.

Although most insurance companies usually refuse to pay for EDTA chelation therapy unless there is a diagnosis of heavy metal toxicity, this historical legal decision opened the doors to greater possibility. It allowed physicians who practice chelation therapy to continue practicing without fear of losing their licenses, and it allowed further research to be done on chelation therapy. As chelation therapy has evolved over the years a new and far more convenient form of EDTA chelation therapy became available, making it possible for anyone to practice chelation therapy at home without having to visit a doctor's office.

I.V. Chelation Versus Oral Chelation

There are two basic forms of EDTA chelation therapy, oral and intravenous (I.V.), and there are two primary forms of EDTA in use, sodium
EDTA and calcium EDTA. Not surprisingly, there is a divergence of
opinion about the relative virtues of these different forms of chelation
therapy. Most of the clinical studies that have been done involve the
intravenous use of sodium EDTA, although this practice is falling out of
favor due to the extensive time commitment that it requires.

An I.V. chelation session using the sodium form of EDTA generally
takes around three or four hours, during which time 1500 mg to 3000
mg of EDTA (plus vitamin C and other nutrients) is administered while
the patient relaxes, socializes, or reads. The I.V. sessions that use the
calcium form of EDTA are much quicker than those using the sodium
form of EDTA, and can be done in just a few minutes. This is because
the calcium form of EDTA stings less when it is administered and can
be injected into the circulatory system much more rapidly.

Traditionally, chelation therapy sessions have been done using the much
slower sodium EDTA method. This was because it was initially thought
that patients should avoid the calcium form of EDTA due to the possibility
of increasing calcium buildup in the circulatory system. However,
although the calcium form of EDTA does add to the bloodstream's supply
of freely-circulating calcium, it appears that this doesn't significantly
increase calcium buildup in the body and calcium EDTA seems to work
as effectively as sodium EDTA. So EDTA chelation therapy sessions
can now be done much more conveniently—in just a few minutes.

The number of I.V. chelation treatments that patients generally require
to treat a particular condition is around twenty to fifty sessions, although
the number of treatments is dependent on the individual's condition.
The best candidates for I.V. chelation are usually people that have
been diagnosed with cardiovascular disease or who are suffering from
heavy metal poisoning, however anyone who wishes to improve their
health stands to benefit from using I.V. chelation therapy because, to
some degree, everyone on this planet is suffering from heavy metal
poisoning.

Many physicians who practice chelation therapy report that oral chelation has some of the benefits of I.V. chelation, although it is not as powerful or as quickly acting. I.V. therapy is much more direct and more powerful because a hundred percent of the EDTA is absorbed into the bloodstream, whereas with oral chelation only around five or ten percent of the dose is absorbed. Because only a small percentage of an oral dose is absorbed into the bloodstream the timing and dosage requirements of the therapy are different. The average dose for oral EDTA is between a thousand and two thousand milligrams, taken twice a day. Oral chelation therapy should be done between meals on an empty stomach, followed by a good multimineral supplement around two hours later. Oral EDTA chelation therapy can be done every day. The most common report that I encounter from healthy people who start oral EDTA chelation therapy is that they now have substantially more energy.

Oral EDTA chelation therapy may actually be the method of choice for people who are simply looking to improve their performance, prevent age-related degenerative diseases, or whose condition does not demand rapid action. Many physicians report that what can be achieved in only a few hours with I.V. chelation may take several weeks or months with oral EDTA chelation. However, the primary benefit of oral chelation is convenience. As long as one follows the proper protocol, and takes a good multimineral supplement several hours after chelating, one can safely chelate at home, without the cost or hassle of a doctor's visit. Oral chelation is very inexpensive. EDTA is about the price of vitamin C, so there really is no reason why everyone shouldn't consider taking it.

Dr. Gordon offers the following metaphor to help distinguish between the relative virtues of different forms of chelation therapy. "To keep it really simple the difference between I.V. and oral chelation is that oral chelation is a little bit like washing your car. It's a good idea and it looks pretty good. I.V. is a little bit like doing a Simoniz®. It does a deeper cleansing, but not everybody can afford to Simoniz® their car," he said.

Although I.V. chelation is more powerful and quickly acting than oral chelation, there may be another benefit to using the oral EDTA chelation besides its convenience—it may help to prevent colon cancer. This often unacknowledged benefit of using EDTA orally is due to an effect within the digestive system known as enterohepatic reuptake, which causes the intestines to reabsorb intestinal bile released by the liver during the digestive process. EDTA prevents the reuptake of this intestinal bile by binding to the heavy metals in it before it can be reabsorbed. This way the bile can be excreted as waste from the body before it forms into the toxic by-products that can lead to colon cancer. By having EDTA present in the digestive system we may be able to help prevent colon cancer.

According to Dr. Gordon, "Everyone would be well-advised to take the oral form of EDTA every day because of the epidemic of colon cancer today. This is due to the interaction between various molecules in the intestinal tract that wind up becoming what we call oxidized bile salts, which can lead to the formation of very toxic substances. These very toxic substances wind up inside ninety-nine percent of all people in America today. When we test people's bowel movements we find carcinogens and mutagens in their feces. People are bathing their poor colons in substances that are so toxic that it's wonder that everybody doesn't get colon cancer. By merely adding EDTA you prevent all of those lipid peroxides and other reactions from going on because you are eliminating the metals that catalyze those bad reactions."

Some supplement companies have recently been marketing EDTA rectal suppositories, claiming that the EDTA in them is a hundred percent absorbed, eliminating the need for I.V. chelation. According to Dr. Gordon, this can't be true because rectal and intestinal absorption are similar, and neither comes close to the hundred percent absorption obtainable through the I.V. route. Advertising EDTA rectal suppositories in this manner is a disservice to people, Dr. Gordon says, because it fools them into thinking that they're getting the benefits of an I.V. chelation when they're not. Also, EDTA rectal suppositories don't prevent blood clots and colon cancer like the oral form does, Dr. Gordon says, because they aren't continuously bathing the intestinal tract with EDTA.

If the EDTA isn't present in the gut then it can't help to prevent the free radical stress on colon cells. In addition, Dr. Gordon points out that if people are interested in lowering the risk of heart attacks, they should take EDTA in conjunction with mucopolysaccharides, like carrageenan, (which is found in red algae, and will be discussed in chapter 3) because taking the two together can help to prevent blood clots in a manner that is greater than the sum total of each on their own. According to my coauthor, the heparin-like effect produced by the combination of EDTA and mucopolysaccarides "makes using aspirin and coumadin for their blood thinning abilities look dangerous and ineffective."

Only the oral form of EDTA can help to tie up the heavy metals that we consume in our food and water, thus helping to prevent them from being absorbed into the body. This is why Dr. Gordon says "the entire concept of rectal EDTA is like putting the cart in front of the horse." According to my coauthor, rectal and oral absorption for most substances are identical. The reason for the rectal administration of some medications is to delay the metabolism of certain substances by the liver, so for some drugs it makes sense to administer it rectally. However, according to Dr. Gordon, "EDTA is not metabolized in the body so there is no logical reason to spend extra money to get EDTA in a rectal preparation. Also, since the main advantage of EDTA administration seems to be in lowering the levels of toxic metals like lead in the body, this means that a long-term treatment of ten to fifteen years is required, and that is a long time to use rectal suppositories."

Another less known form of chelation therapy involves simply soaking one's body in EDTA by adding it to one's bath water. According to studies done by Andrew Sincock, microscopic aquatic animals called rotifers raised in an environment with EDTA lived approximately fifty percent longer than a control group.[12] The EDTA extended both the lifespan and the reproductive period of the rotifers. This research has inspired my coauthor to begin developing EDTA bath therapy formulas, and has been using EDTA in this manner himself with good results, such as improved skin tone.

Is EDTA Chelation Therapy Being Deliberately Suppressed?

Despite the fact that a review of the scientific literature supports the assertion that EDTA chelation therapy can have numerous beneficial effects on people's health, the official position from the American Heart Association (AHA) on chelation—according to their Web site—is that "there is no scientific evidence that demonstrates any benefit from this form of therapy in the treatment of arteriosclerotic heart disease."

Neither the American Medical Association (AMA) or the FDA acknowledge EDTA chelation therapy as a treatment for heart disease or for many of its other demonstrated health benefits. Organizations like the AHA and the AMA, which say that EDTA chelation therapy is ineffective for treating cardiovascular disease, ignore the mountains of evidence that would lead one to believe otherwise, and they generally quote two studies to support their position—a Danish study done in 1991 and 1992, and a New Zealand study done in 1994.

In 1992 researchers in Denmark published results from a clinical trial of a hundred and fifty-three patients with intermittent claudication,[13] an atherosclerosis-related condition characterized by pain and weakness in the legs that is exacerbated by walking. The researchers were a group of cardiovascular surgeons who openly admitted their opposition to chelation therapy. According to a statement by Dr. Claude Lenfant on the U.S. Department of Health and Human Services Web site, "the scientists noted that the results reflect "the well-known phenomenon of spontaneous improvement,"—commonly known as the "placebo effect"—in which patients feel or function better for no reason other than that they are being treated or observed. They concluded that EDTA chelation therapy had no beneficial effect among the patients in the trial."

Then, two years later, in 1994, a group of researchers—also cardio-vascular surgeons—at Otago Medical School in New Zealand published results from a similar clinical study of thirty-two patients also with intermittent claudication.[14] Fifteen of the patients underwent EDTA chelation therapy, and seventeen patients were given a placebo of saline solution. Walking distance was used as the major measure of improvement. At the end of the treatment period, sixty percent of the chelation group showed an increase in walking distance. However, fifty-nine percent of the saline or placebo group also demonstrated an improvement. According to the U.S. Department of Health and Human Services Web site, "As with the Danish study, these results again provide a classic illustration of the placebo effect—that is, improvement that springs from the mere fact of being treated, rather than from the results of the specific treatment itself. The New Zealand scientists therefore concluded, like the Danish researchers, that EDTA chelation therapy has no significant beneficial effects."

Statements from these highly influential organizations, which claim that the benefits that people experience with EDTA chelation therapy are simply due to the power of the placebo effect (i.e., the power of one's mind to measurably improve health, which many conventional medical authorities also tend to devalue) fail to mention that the Danish studies were actually criticized by the Danish Committee for Investigation into Scientific Dishonesty.[15] They were criticized because of a lack of improper randomization and double-blinding, as well as for a premature breaking of the blinding code, which, basically, amounted to a deliberate bias.

Although the study was alleged to have been conducted in a double-blind manner (meaning that neither the patients or the researchers were supposed to know who received EDTA and who received a placebo), the researchers later revealed that they broke the code before the post-treatment final evaluation. Not only did the researchers themselves know before the end of the study who was receiving EDTA and who was receiving a placebo, they had also revealed this information to many of the test subjects. Before the study was over more than sixty-four percent of the subjects were aware of which treatment they had received. From an ethical and scientific standpoint this is a highly questionable procedure, precisely because of the very effect that the researchers claimed to be measuring—the placebo effect, which changes the results in a measurable way.

If these research methods weren't unscientific and unethical enough, according to Drs. Elmer Cranton and James Frackelton in *A Textbook on EDTA Chelation Therapy*, "one important aspect of the Danish study is the startling fact that the patients who were given EDTA were much sicker than the patients treated with a placebo. Therefore, the improvements the EDTA group made were harder earned and more significant."[16]

The statistics used in this study have also been called into question. According to Cranton and Frackelton, the plus or minus thirty-eight meters standard deviations for EDTA patients versus the plus or minus two hundred sixty-six meters standard deviations for the placebo group represents an enormous variation in walking capacity that is heavily biased in favor of the placebo group. These standard deviations imply that some placebo patients must have walked half a mile before stopping. This means that the placebo group's claudication was markedly less severe, and the EDTA group was much more severely diseased—so the design of the study was obviously biased against EDTA chelation from the outset.

However, when the six-month study was completed the mean maximal walking distance in the EDTA group increased by 51.3 percent, from 119 to 180 meters, while the mean maximal walking distance in the placebo group increased only 23.6 percent, from 157 to 194 meters. The chelation group's improvement was therefore more than twice as great as the placebo group's, even though the chelation group was significantly sicker at the outset. According to Cranton and Frackelton, "This is a positive study, supporting the usefulness of EDTA chelation. The authors' published negative conclusions are not supported by the data."

The results from the New Zealand research were examined by two independent statisticians, and it was concluded that this study also actually supported the efficacy of EDTA. According to Cranton and Frackelton "Absolute walking distance in the EDTA group increased by 25.9 percent; while in the placebo group, it increased by 14.8 percent. The difference was not considered statistically significant. The study, however had only 17 subjects in the placebo group. One of the placebo patients was what the statisticians call an "outlier," whose results differ strikingly from everyone else in the group. This patient's walking distance increased by almost 500 meters. All of the statistical gain in the placebo group was due to this one individual's progress. Without him, the placebo group's distance actually decreased. This illustrates the perils of a small study. The 25 percent gain in the EDTA group compared to no gain in the placebo group would have been very significant statistically."

However, as a result of these undeserved official denouncements of chelation therapy, many people have come to dismiss it as if it were some kind of New Age snake oil. Not surprisingly, those who believe in the efficacy of EDTA chelation therapy tend to support the notion that this misinformation about the therapy was deliberately spread by these official organizations because the patent on EDTA ran out and the pharmaceutical companies can no longer profit from its sale.

Could this be true? Cardiovascular surgery is an enormously profitable enterprise and the medical community would lose a substantial portion of its profits if an inexpensive and equally effective treatment were to be offered as an alternative. Coronary artery bypass surgery alone is an 18.4 billion dollar a year industry. Many people believe that this is the primary reason why EDTA chelation therapy is not more widely practiced.

Support for this point of view comes from a study where sixty-five patients on a waiting list for coronary artery bypass surgery were treated with EDTA chelation therapy and the symptoms in eighty-nine percent improved so much that they were able to cancel their surgery.[17] While I don't wish to second-guess the motives of titanic medical organizations like the AMA and the FDA, I do want to point out that the consequences of suppressing this effective and inexpensive treatment could be costing us countless lives.

There may be other reasons why EDTA chelation therapy isn't more widely practiced. In addition to these misleading denouncements by official medical organizations, the mechanism of action isn't well understood. Since chelation therapy isn't dissolving away cardiovascular blockages as was originally thought, it remains a bit of a mystery why it lowers blood pressure, improves circulation, and generally improves cardiovascular health.

Understanding the mechanism of EDTA's action may mean accepting the revelation that everyone is suffering from some degree of lead toxicity. This is something that many people may not want to admit— certainly not the health insurance companies or the petroleum industry. In the next chapter we'll look more closely at heavy metal toxicity and how EDTA chelation therapy can be an essential tool in detoxifying our bodies from this overly polluted world that we have created.

Chapter 2

REMOVING ENVIRONMENTAL TOXINS

AND

HEAVY METALS

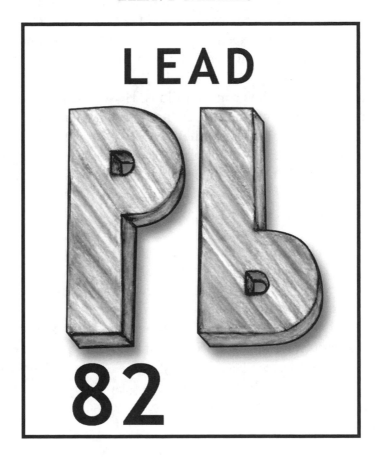

The degree of health or illness that people experience in their life generally depends upon the balance that they achieve between the toxic and protective forces in their bodies. It is as though one's state of wellness is the result of a battle between the forces of "good and evil" played out on a biochemical level. The malicious demons that threaten our health and well-being come in the form of heavy metal environmental contaminants and the angelic protectors that gloriously come to our rescue are the cells in our body's detoxification system— aided by whatever we can do to assist them. In this context, EDTA chelation therapy is like a band of angels sent from the Heavens to battle for the improved health of your body.

What are Heavy Metals?

Heavy metals are natural components of the Earth's crust and they cannot be degraded or destroyed. The primary heavy metals that we are referring to in this chapter are lead, mercury, aluminum, arsenic, cadmium, and nickel, but the term "heavy metal" refers to any metallic chemical element that has a relatively high density and is toxic or poisonous at relatively low concentrations. Heavy metals have a higher molecular weight than most substances and are characterized by a specific gravity that is at least five times that of water. They have been widely used in industry since the 1800s and are now common environmental contaminants. In other words, since the 1800s humans have assisted in the mass migration of heavy metals from the earth's crust into our air, water, food, and bodies.

Most heavy metals are extremely toxic to the body because they tend to combine with and inhibit the metabolic functioning of particular enzymes. They are especially dangerous because they tend to accumulate in the body over time. This means that there is an increase in the body's concentration of the heavy metal as time goes by, compared to the chemical's concentration in the environment. Heavy metals tend to accumulate in our bodies because they are taken up and stored faster than they can generally be excreted. They also tend to accumulate in ecosystems for the same reason, which compounds the problem even further.

Living organisms require trace amounts of some heavy metals—such as cobalt, copper, manganese, and zinc—but excessive levels can be detrimental to the organism. Other heavy metals such as mercury, lead and cadmium have no known beneficial effect on any living organisms, and their accumulation over time in the human body can cause serious illness. Even minute amounts of heavy metals can have severe physiological or neurological effects and this is precisely why EDTA is such a godsend.

EDTA eagerly binds with heavy metals in the circulatory system and quickly whisks them out of the body. Three of the heavy metals that EDTA has the greatest affinity with are lead, mercury, and cadmium. This means that whenever an EDTA molecule encounters one of these heavy metals in the body during chelation therapy it will hastily drop whatever metal or mineral that it is already bound to and eagerly bind to the lead, mercury, or cadmium on its journey out of the body. EDTA seems to especially love lead. When EDTA encounters lead it's like Cinderella meeting her prince. Lead and EDTA are like soul-mates; they grab hold of each other and don't let go—which is good news for us.

What Is Lead?

Lead is a bluish-white heavy metal that has been used by human beings for at least seven thousand years. It's distributed widely and it's easy to extract from the Earth. Lead is also easy to work with because it is highly malleable and easy to melt. Ancient alchemists thought that lead was the oldest of all metals and they associated it with the planet Saturn. A form of lead poisoning known as saturnine gout takes its name from this association. Saturn was the dark, gloomy, and irritable god who ate his own children. Some ancient Romans noticed similarities between symptoms of this disorder and the irritable god, and named the disease after him.

Lead is soft yet very durable. Some lead pipes that bear the insignia of Roman emperors are still in service to this day. Lead is also highly toxic to human beings. It inhibits enzymes in many biochemical pathways, and because lead and zinc are so closely related to each other chemically, our bodies will actually plug lead into key enzyme functions that normally zinc would have fulfilled. This can cause a multitude of health problems.

Some historians and toxicologists believe that the fall of the Roman empire was actually accelerated by the chronic lead poisoning experienced by the ruling classes. Lead influenced many areas of Roman life. It made up pipes, paints, dishes, cosmetics, coins, and bullets. The Romans had water conducted through lead plumbing and they drank wine from goblets which had a partial lead composition. Eventually, as a host of mysterious ailments became more common, some Romans began to suspect a connection between lead and these illnesses. However, the

Roman culture's habits didn't change, and some historians believe that many among the Roman aristocracy suffered from lead poisoning.

The symptoms of lead poisoning include neurological problems, such as reduced intelligence, and numerous researchers have confirmed a direct link between early lead exposure in children and serious learning disabilities.[1] Some of the other symptoms of lead poisoning include gastrointestinal problems, such as abdominal pain, nausea, constipation, diarrhea, poor appetite, and weight loss. Other associated effects include kidney complications, reproductive problems, anemia, irritability, excess lethargy or hyperactivity, insomnia, headache, and, in extreme cases, seizure and coma.

As a result of reckless and misguided human activity over the past two hundred years, studies indicate that there is now so much lead circulating in our biosphere that it is simply impossible to live on this planet and avoid exposure to it.[2,3] Although dedicated environmental groups are working to reduce lead levels in the biosphere, the levels of lead in our environment are still catastrophically high, and rising lead levels in the body—below what most physicians consider "lead poisoning"—have nonetheless been linked to numerous diseases, such as the formation of cataracts in the eye[4] and an increased risk of cardiovascular disease. [5]

In other words, the central message of this book can now be summed up in a single sentence: Researchers have confirmed that everyone on this planet is suffering from lead poisoning and medical experts agree that the only effective way to treat lead poisoning is chelation therapy.

What About Other Heavy Metals?

Besides lead, two of the other most prevalent heavy metals in our environment are mercury and cadmium. Mercury is a silvery transition metal. It is one of only five elements that are liquid at room temperature, but chemical variations of the element can also exist in a gaseous form. The major natural source of mercury is the degassing of the Earth's crust, emissions from volcanoes, and the evaporation from natural bodies of water. Mercury is a toxic substance which has no known function in human biochemistry and does not occur naturally in living organisms. Mercury poisoning is associated with tremors, gingivitis, spontaneous abortion, and developmental changes in young children. It is also associated with psychological changes and causes damage to the brain and the central nervous system.

The zany character in Lewis Carrol's children's book *Alice in Wonderland*, who threw literature's most memorable tea party—the Mad Hatter—was based upon the caricatures of actual hat makers in England during the 1800s who developed psychiatric disorders as a result of working with a mercury solution that was commonly used during the process of turning fur into felt. During this process the hat makers would breathe in the mercury fumes, and the problem was exacerbated by the poor ventilation in most of the workshops. This led to an accumulation of mercury in the hat makers' bodies, which resulted in symptoms such as slurred speech, memory loss, trembling, loss of coordination, depression, and anxiety—as well as inspiring the phrase "mad as a hatter."

While the hat making industry has long since banned this dangerous practice, the worldwide mining of mercury has lead to its presence in the atmosphere, and the usage of mercury in industrial processes, as well as in various products—such as thermometers, barometers, and batteries—is widespread. Believe it or not, mercury is also used widely in dentistry as an amalgam for fillings and by the pharmaceutical industry as a preservative in vaccines (which we will discuss more in chapter 4). Natural biological processes can cause methylated forms of mercury to form and concentrate in living organisms—especially fish—and these forms of mercury can accumulate in living tissue over a million-fold. These highly toxic organic compounds of mercury—known as monomethylmercury and dimethylmercury—are extremely toxic and are known to cause serious neurological disorders. Like lead, mercury is a potent neurotoxin, and elevated blood mercury levels have led to retardation and deformities in children.

Fish and shellfish have a natural tendency to concentrate mercury in their bodies, often in the form of methylmercury. Species of fish that are high on the food chain—such as swordfish, king mackerel, and albacore tuna—contain higher concentrations of mercury than others. This is because mercury is stored in the muscles of fish, and when a predatory fish makes a meal of another fish it then assumes the entire body burden of mercury in the consumed fish. Since fish are less efficient at eliminating methylmercury than they are at accumulating it, the concentrations of methylmercury in the muscle tissue of the fish tend to increase over time. This means that species that are high up on the food chain amass body burdens of mercury that can be ten times higher, or more, than the species that they consume.

However, even with all that unhealthy mercury in our fish, it is worth noting that there may also be a danger in eliminating fish from one's diet—especially cold water oily fish, such as salmon, herring, mackerel, anchovies, and sardines, as they are rich in anti-inflammatory, essential omega fatty acids. In general, people who regularly include cold water fish in their diets have significantly longer lifespans and less cardiovascular disease than people who don't. Luckily, these important essential fatty acids can also be obtained from refined fish oil supplements that remove mercury and other contaminants, as well as from hemp and flax seed oil.

Cadmium is a soft and malleable, bluish-white, transition metal that can easily be cut with a knife. It is used in batteries, pigments, as a stabilizer for plastics, and as a barrier to control nuclear fission. Like lead, cadmium derives its toxicological properties from its chemical similarity to zinc. Once cadmium is absorbed it generally remains stored in the body for many years. Long-term exposure to cadmium is associated with kidney problems. High exposure can lead to obstructive lung disease and has been linked to lung cancer. Studies show that cadmium may also cause osteoporosis and other bone defects, as well as increased blood pressure and other health problems.

The giant dark clouds of lead, mercury, and cadmium particles that have descended upon our precious and fragile world are a truly serious problem indeed—but the problem looms larger still.

The Biosphere 2 Project

From September 26, 1991 to September 26, 1993 a courageous group of eight men and women—including the late UCLA longevity researcher Roy Walford—set off on a path of ecological discovery in the Oracle, Arizona desert called the Biosphere 2 project. This visionary project lead to the creation of the largest artificial, self-sustaining ecosystem ever built and was truly a masterpiece of human engineering. For two years and twenty minutes, inside a completely sealed, glass-enclosed 3.15 acre environment—composed of miniature replicas of all the earth's environments, and housing 3,800 species of plants and animals, designed to function together as a single system—these eight people had to grow all their own vegetables, raise all their own livestock, and live so that a hundred percent of their waste was recycled. In other words, the animals and plants in Biosphere 2 had to produce all of their own biological resources without polluting one another out of existence. Biosphere 2 was the most tightly sealed structure ever built by human beings and no air, water, or food could be brought in from the outside once the project began.[6,7]

I interviewed John Allen, who largely designed the Biosphere 2 project, for one of my earlier books and we became good friends. I spent a lot of time with John and several of the Biosphere 2 crew members after their two year mission. All of the people involved in the project stressed to me how important ecological awareness was while they were living within the hermetically-sealed environment—because every single molecule of air and water, and all nutrients within Biosphere 2, had to be completely recycled. Living inside such a small closed environment it becomes obvious rather quickly that the waste that people flush down their toilet will wind up in everyone's drinking water a few days later if its not a hundred percent biodegradable, as all the water and resources in Biosphere 2 are so quickly recycled. For this reason, all farming had to be organic and no pesticides or toxins of any kind could be used.

Now, in larger sense, the same sort of process is going on with the planetary biosphere that we call home, only it's not as obvious. The plants and animals on this planet create all of the nutrients necessary to sustain life from one another's waste, and any chemical toxins or heavy metals that we release into our atmosphere or oceans quickly finds its way into the air we breathe and the water we drink because the biosphere is a single system. This is why you find the flame retardant used in American children's pajamas in the fatty flesh of animals that live in both the Antarctic and Arctic Circle. Once one grasps this elementary principle, it becomes clear that by polluting our environment we're seriously poisoning ourselves. After one realizes this it's hard not to become angry at the people who are spewing toxic waste into the air that we all have to breathe and into the water that we all have to drink. When major industries release toxic waste into our biosphere it's analogous to having inconsiderate people pee in a public pool that we all share—only worse.

Life on a Poisoned Planet

Every single human being on planet Earth is suffering from some degree of exposure to toxic chemicals and to heavy metal poisoning. In America alone, more than six billion pounds of chemical toxins are released every year. Through industrialization and the burning of fossil fuels, our land, air and water has become ubiquitously contaminated and polluted. In the every day course of our lives, simply breathing, eating, drinking, and cleaning ourselves causes us to accumulate dangerous toxins and heavy metals in our bodies. The primary sources of these heavy metals are air emissions from coal-burning plants and other industrial facilities, waste incinerators, process wastes from mining and industry, pesticides and wood preservatives, fertilizer, and old household plumbing with lead pipes or lead-based house paints.

An article by David Ewing Duncan in the October, 2006 issue of *National Geographic* magazine entitled "The Pollution Within" documented with disturbing detail how many of the toxic chemicals of modern life are building up in our bodies and staying there for years, where they may be causing a wide range of mysterious illnesses.[8] When the writer of the article had a chemical analysis done of his blood—which checked for 320 toxic chemicals commonly found in our environment—he discovered dangerously high levels of PCBs, pesticides, dioxins, and heavy metals in his body. After eating a single meal of halibut and swordfish, caught in the San Francisco Bay, the author's blood-mercury level more than doubled. The central message of the article was that there wasn't anything terribly unique about this journalist that put him more at risk for absorbing toxins than the average person, and that our environment is thoroughly contaminated by dangerous chemicals and heavy metals.

According to the Congressional Office of Technology Assessment, there are currently six hundred thousand toxic-waste contamination sites in the United States alone. Of these, the Environmental Protection Agency has proposed fewer than nine hundred for cleanup and approximately nineteen thousand others are under review. The impact that toxic waste is having on our environment is difficult to calculate, but it's pretty clear that all these toxins and heavy metals being released into the environment isn't good news for fragile organisms like us.

For example, an important study at the Tulane University School of Public Health demonstrated that the average blood level of lead found among Americans is high enough to increase the likelihood of cardiovascular diseases, such as strokes and heart attacks.[9] Another study by Debra Schaumberg at Harvard University showed that the higher the percentage of lead that there is in the bones the more likely people are to develop cataracts in their eyes.[10]

Heavy metal pollution in the United States is largely a result of earlier uses, such as burning leaded gasoline for fuel. Lead from gasoline accounts for eighty to ninety percent of all existing environmental lead contamination. Because lead is a chemical element it cannot be degraded or transformed into another substance and it is extremely difficult to clean up after dispersal into the environment. Even if all heavy metal production were to stop today, enough heavy metals have already been released into our environment to continue causing serious problems for generations to come.

Heavy metals are simply impossible to avoid on this planet. Arsenic, lead, and mercury are in the air we breathe. There is aluminum in much of our cookware and cadmium is in many of our refined foods. As noted earlier in this chapter, seafood is loaded with mercury and a number of vaccines actually use mercury as a preservative. According to the National Autism Association, children are twenty-seven times more likely to develop autism after they've been exposed to mercury-containing vaccines. (The relationship between autism and heavy metal poisoning will be explored in chapter 4 on chelation therapy and mental health.)

More than two hundred twenty-five million Americans even have mercury-amalgam dental fillings—which were actually declared a hazardous substance by the Environmental Protection Agency in

1989—in their teeth that are exposing them to microscopic particles and mercury vapors every time they chew. We all live in a soup of toxins and heavy metals that are continuously threatening our health and well-being.

This is a serious problem because heavy metals are everywhere. According to Dr. Gordon, "Every blade of grass and every plant is loaded with lead, mercury, and cadmium from the fallout of the particulate matter. It's in the air that we breathe and it goes directly into our bodies. We find that mercury—from the burning of coal in China—is actually present in birds on Mount Washington at a ten thousand foot elevation. We can find this in the birds because it's in their diet. It's coating all the foodstuff that everybody eats. All these heavy metals are impossible to avoid. The Earth has become so totally polluted that every person today is walking around with lead, mercury, and cadmium in their body. They're in every human being we test today."

When Clair Patterson, from the California Institute of Technology, carefully drilled down into the ice cores of the Arctic and Antarctic to find out when the lead levels in our biosphere began to rise, he had to put his researchers into special tightly sealed suits—as if they were going into outer space—so that they wouldn't contaminate the ice core samples.[11] This is because one drop of human sweat, a drop from a nasal secretion, a flake of dead skin, or a piece of hair, is so filled with lead that it would have contaminated his study.

Even Our Homes Aren't Safe

Dangerous toxins and pollutants are everywhere. Even our homes aren't safe. The average American home contains about a hundred pounds of hazardous chemicals and waste. According to David Ewing Duncan's October, 2006 *National Geographic* article mentioned above, our homes are overflowing with toxic chemicals that seep into our bodies. For example, polybrominated diphenyl (PBDEs)—toxic chemicals used as flame retardants and known to cause developmental problems in laboratory animals—are found in many household appliances, such as hair dryers, telephones, televisions, and computers. They are also commonly found in fabrics, pillows, carpets, and chair cushions.

Although some of the more toxic pesticides, such as DDT, have been banned, the list of dangerous pesticides currently in use is enough to frighten Stephen King. Many of our agricultural products are literally soaked with an exotic array of scary chemicals that are known to cause health problems. We have literally poisoned much of our food supply and this is why it is so important to buy organic produce. Pesticides can also be found in common household items like antimicrobial soap and pet flea collars.

Polychlorinated biphenyls (PCBs) are an unnatural mixture of different highly toxic chlorinated compounds that were used as coolants and lubricants in electrical equipment. Because of evidence that they accumulate in the environment and can cause harmful health effects, in 1977 the manufacture of PCBs was halted in the U.S.—although they are still being released from hazardous waste sites. PCBs do not break down easily and remain in the environment for many years. They can be found in fish and game from contaminated areas. The effects of PCBs include cancer and liver damage in laboratory animals.

Polycarbonate plastics, which are used to manufacture some plastic bottles, can also be a huge problem. These types of plastics utilize a compound called bisphenol A—which is used to help keep some plastic drinking water bottles rigid. Bisphenol A is a synthetic estrogen that mimics the female hormone once it enters the human body and it is known to cause reproductive harm to the human fetus. Bisphenol A can be found in many drinking water bottles and even in some baby bottles.

Perflurooctane acid (PFOA) is used in some fabrics to make them stain resistant and on some frying pans to create a nonstick surface, even though it is known to cause cancer in laboratory animals. It's impossible to avoid PFOA and another related compound, perfluorooctane sulfonate (PFOS), which although no longer used, also pervades the global environment and can be found in our air, water, and food.

Dioxins are a group of hundreds of highly toxic chemicals that are formed as an unintentional byproduct of many industrial processes involving chlorine, such as waste incineration and pesticide manufacturing.

Dioxins build up in the fats of animals and plants that are raised in contaminated areas and they are sometimes found in fatty meats.

Phthalates are used in many body lotions to give them the proper consistency. They are found in a number of household items, such as in vinyl, where it is used to improve flexibility. They can be found in deodorants, soaps, hair sprays, extension cords, and shower curtains— even though laboratory studies have shown that they can cause problems with male sexual development.

In other words, toxic chemicals and heavy metals are so ubiquitous and so pervasive in every environment on this planet that we're literally swimming in a soup of this stuff. It is estimated there are currently over a hundred thousand toxic chemicals in our environment with over twenty-five percent of these known to be carcinogenic. Significant quantities of around sixty to eighty pesticides are present in the food being consumed by most Americans. Fifty percent of the water supplies in the United States are contaminated with toxic chemicals. Over six hundred thousand babies born in America are known to have mercury toxicity, and the average American today has at least forty carcinogens and forty-to-fifty neurotoxic substances in their blood stream at all times. Our bodies are simply soaked with PBDEs, PCBs, bisphenols, PFOAs, PFOSs, dioxins, phthalates, and heavy metal particles—so everyone's health is compromised to some extent as a result.

How Does the Body Deal With Toxic Substances?

Our body handles toxins by either neutralizing, transforming, or eliminating them. The body's primary defense against metabolic poisoning is carried out by the liver and the kidneys, although it also uses natural chelators, such as vitamin C, to help remove heavy metals from the circulatory system. The kidneys filter wastes from the blood and excrete them, along with water, as urine. The liver is responsible for the production of bile which is stored in the gallbladder and released when required for the digestion of fats. The liver has also evolved mechanisms to convert fat-soluble chemicals into water-soluble chemicals so that they may then be excreted from the body via watery fluids such as bile and urine. We also clear toxins through sweating, from heat or exercise.

Over millions of years the liver has evolved sophisticated mechanisms for breaking down toxic substances and it helps to transform many of these toxic substances into harmless agents. The liver is the gateway into the body and in this polluted world its easy to see how its detoxification systems can easily become overloaded. Thousands of chemicals have been added to our food and hundreds of chemicals have been identified in our drinking water. Plants are sprayed with toxic pesticides, animals are injected with antibiotics and hormones, and a significant amount of our food is genetically engineered and heavily processed.

All this can lead to the destruction of delicate vitamins and minerals, which are needed for the detoxification pathways in the liver. When the liver tries to cope with all these toxic chemicals in our environment and our processed foods, it can easily become overwhelmed. Drugs, artificial chemicals, and pesticides are metabolized by enzyme pathways inside the liver cells, and heavy metals are particularly difficult for the body to excrete because they can not be broken down or metabolized. This is why they tend to accumulate in the body over time.

Praise the heavens that we have help in this process! In addition to the body's natural defense against toxins, numerous methods have been developed by open-minded healthcare professionals for eliminating toxic substances from the body and assisting the body's natural detoxification process—such as modifying one's diet and adding certain herbs, as well as colonic cleansing, juice fasting, and saunas. In extreme cases, detoxification needs to be achieved through technological assistance, such as by dialysis. But, by and far, the best all-around defense against the dangers of toxic metals appears to be chelation therapy combined with strong nutritional support.

Aiding the Body's Defense Against Toxins

In addition to using EDTA chelation therapy to help rid the body of dangerous heavy metals, there are a number of herbal and nutritional substances that can aid in the body's defense against environmental toxins, such pesticides, PCBs, phthalates, and dioxins. Dr. Gordon also recommends chelating farm animals to help remove heavy metals from their systems before using them for meat or dairy products. Some of the most important nutritional and herbal supplements with properties that help to detoxify the body are vitamin C, selenium, garlic, MSM, fiber, and D-ribose.

Vitamin C

Vitamin C, or ascorbic acid, is an essential nutrient. This means that it can not be synthesized by the body and must be supplied through the diet. Somewhere in our recent evolutionary past as primates we lost our ability to synthesize ascorbic acid, like most other mammals, so we must obtain it through the food that we eat or the supplements that we take. Vitamin C is a powerful antioxidant, a chemical that prevents the oxidative degradation of other chemicals and helps to neutralize dangerous free radicals in the body.

Free radicals are highly reactive atoms or molecules with unpaired electrons and they can cause substantial oxidative damage to the body. This can lead to a number of chronic diseases, such as heart disease and cancer, and many gerontologists think that free radical damage is one of the primary causes of aging. Because free radicals are necessary for normal metabolism, the body uses antioxidants, such as vitamins C and E, to minimize free radical-induced damage. Vitamin C's antioxidant properties also help to cut down the damage done by environmental toxins and it sometimes acts as chelator to help remove heavy metals.

Dosages of 3000 milligrams of vitamin C per day have been shown to remove aluminum from brain cells[12]—which could help to prevent Alzheimer's Disease and other neurological disorders[13]—and numerous studies have demonstrated that vitamin C can help to prevent cancer[14,15] and heart disease.[16] It's important to take enough vitamin C to reap the benefits that have been revealed in scientific studies without upsetting one's digestive system, as too much vitamin C can cause bowel intolerance—although this problem can virtually be eliminated by using buffered forms of vitamin C.

Nutritionists are quick to point out that the U.S. Recommended Daily Allowance for vitamin C is egregiously outdated, and only provides enough of the essential nutrient to prevent deficiency diseases, such as scurvy. Studies show that an optimal dose of vitamin C is around 2000 milligrams per day in divided doses.[17] Obtaining these levels of vitamin C from diet alone is close to impossible, so it's important to take supplements if one is interested in obtaining optimal health.

There are different forms of vitamin C and the body responds to them in different ways. It's important to take a form of vitamin C that is easily absorbed and well tolerated by the digestive system. Vitamin C that is composed of mineral ascorbates has a high bioavailability and many people report that this form of vitamin C tends to be more easily tolerated by the digestive system than other forms of ascorbic acid. Sometimes plant pigments called bioflavonoids and vitamin C metabolites are added to vitamin C in order to increase its bioavailability.

Vitamin therapy for optimal health is too big of a topic for this book, but it's important to point out that vitamins work best when taken together. Vitamins work synergistically with each other and it's important to take them all. For more information about vitamin therapy see my previous book *Mavericks of Medicine*.

Selenium

Another important nutrient that can help the body to detoxify from environmental toxins is selenium. Selenium is a trace mineral and a chemical element that is essential for proper health, although it is only required in small amounts, measured in micrograms. The body incorporates selenium into proteins to make what are called "selenoproteins"—which are important antioxidant enzymes. The antioxidant properties of some selenoproteins help to prevent cellular damage from free radicals, while other selenoproteins help regulate thyroid function and play a role in the immune system.

Selenium is also known to have protective effects against mercury poisoning and helps to reduce the negative effects of mercury exposure. There is an unusually high bonding affinity between mercury and selenium. As a result of this high bonding affinity, selenium sequesters mercury and reduces its biological availability.[18] In other words, mercury and selenium stick to one another like magnets, and mercury that is bound to selenium can't bind to anything else. In one study, Japanese researchers found that by adding selenium to the diets of birds it "gave complete protection" from large amounts of mercury.

Because mercury poisoning is ubiquitous among the human species, it is extremely important to have proper levels of selenium in the body. Although selenium is an essential nutrient, too much of it can be toxic. However getting enough selenium can sometimes be difficult to obtain from one's diet alone. Selenium occurs primarily in plant foods such as corn, wheat, and soybean, and the content of this important trace mineral in one's food depends upon the selenium content of the soil where plants are grown, which can vary dramatically around the world. The recommended supplemental dosage of selenium is between 100 and 200 micrograms per day.[19]

Garlic

Garlic is a perennial plant closely related to the onion and leek. Like corn and bananas, garlic is a cultigen. This means that it does not grow in the wild and is thought to have been bred in cultivation, descended from a related species that grows wild in southwestern Asia. Garlic has been used throughout all of recorded history for both culinary and medicinal purposes.

When garlic is crushed or finely chopped it yields a powerful antibiotic called allicin and an anti-fungal compound called phytoncide. It also contains enzymes, vitamin B, minerals, and flavonoids. Research with garlic indicates that it has a number of medicinal uses. It may help lower blood pressure, homocysteine levels, and inhibit atherosclerosis.[20, 21] Garlic has been shown to diminish platelet aggregation and lower low density lipoprotein carrying cholesterol. It may have some cancer-fighting properties because it is high in a substance called "diallyl sulphide," which is believed to be an anticarcinogen.[22] Garlic supplementation in rats, along with a high protein diet, has been shown to boost testosterone levels.[23] It has even been shown to help prevent and treat the common cold.[24] Folklore suggests that its effective against mosquitoes and vampires too.

But, perhaps most importantly, garlic helps to detoxify our bodies from environmental toxins. A number of studies have shown that garlic helps to detoxify carcinogenic chemicals and helps to prevent against cancer, as well as liver and kidney disease.[25] In addition to having antioxidant, antibiotic, and antifungal properties, garlic stimulates an immune response by the body. It increases macrophage activity and the number of killer cells in the immune system.

A 2000 study at Annamalai University in India demonstrated that compounds in garlic can protect against the toxic oxidative damage caused by a carcinogen known as MNNG (N-methyl-N'-nitro-N-nitrosoguanidine) and it significantly decreased the formation of toxic metabolic compounds.[26] The study also showed that garlic improved antioxidant levels and increased the number of detoxifying enzymes in the stomach and liver.

While the benefits of garlic are well-known, eating a lot of garlic may not always be practical or socially desirable. The strong odor of garlic on one's breath is often a deterring factor in eating enough of it to reap its medicinal benefits. There are deodorized garlic supplements available, but one has to be careful to obtain a supplement that also contains garlic's medicinal properties and there is some skepticism about whether this is even possible.

The most potent medicinal compound derived from garlic is allicin and the chemistry of this antibiotic is complex. Allicin is not present in natural garlic and is only released when garlic is crushed. Because allicin is unstable and breaks down quickly, its important to find a supplement that has standardized allicin levels. Unfortunately, it is allicin that actually gives garlic its strong odor so many manufacturers standardize the amount of allicin in their product. Alliin is a precursor to allicin, which means that the body needs to convert the alliin into allicin, and this may not be as effective as consuming garlic with high allicin levels.

The recommended dose of garlic is determined by the alliin or allicin levels that the product contains. Research indicates that the daily dosage of a garlic product should provide at least ten milligrams of alliin or a total allicin potential of four thousand micrograms. This dosage equates to roughly one to four cloves of fresh garlic per day.

MSM

MSM (methylsulfonylmethane) is a sulfur compound that occurs naturally in the human body and is found in fruits, vegetables, seafood, and meat. The concentration of MSM in the body tends to decrease with age, and some research suggests that there is a minimum concentration of the sulfur compound that must be maintained in the body in order to preserve normal function and structure. After ingestion, MSM gives up its sulfur to the essential amino acids cysteine, methionine, and other serum proteins in the body. It eventually finds its way into the collagen of skin, joints and blood vessels, and is also incorporated into the keratin of hair and nails.

Many people use MSM supplements for their ability to ameliorate a variety of allergic responses, as well as the pain associated with systemic inflammatory disorders, especially in the joints. MSM reduces inflammation and it is also essential for detoxification. Like fresh garlic, MSM provides a bioavailable dietary source of sulfur, which can help to protect the body against environmental toxins. Sulfur is a vital part of our body's waste management system, and if we don't get enough of it our bodies are not able to release some of their waste. In addition to providing sulfur for the body's waste management system, MSM makes the cell walls more permeable and more elastic. This allows for an easier chemical exchange through the cell wall, and this enables your cells and tissues to release toxins that have built up over the years.

Although MSM is naturally found in many foods, refinement and processing methods often remove much of the MSM, along with vital vitamins and minerals, so supplementation is recommended. A daily dose of 1000 to 3000 milligrams, in divided doses, has been suggested, and some evidence indicates that the benefits of MSM are enhanced when taken with vitamin C.

The Cleansing Power of Fiber

Dietary fibers are the indigestible portion of plant foods that move food through the digestive system, absorbing water and cleansing the intestinal tract. Chemically, dietary fiber consists of non-starch polysaccharides and several other plant components, such as cellulose, waxes, and pectins.

Sources of dietary fiber are usually divided according to whether or not they are water-soluble. Both types of fiber are present in all plant foods—with varying degrees of each according to the plant's characteristics—and, although they're indigestible, they are an important part of the digestive process. Both forms of fiber possess water-attracting properties that help to increase bulk, softening stools and shortening the transit time of food through the intestinal tract. Soluble fiber also undergoes active metabolic processing due to fermentation in the intestines, and this yields end-products with broad and significant health effects.

One of the most versatile sources of dietary fiber is the husk of seeds from psyllium grain, a fiber source with clinically demonstrated properties of lowering blood cholesterol when it is included in one's diet. Psyllium seed husk is thirty-four percent insoluble fiber and sixty-six percent soluble fiber, providing an optimal division of both types that make it a valuable food additive.

Another valuable source of fiber comes from rice. Rice bran is the most nutrient dense food that we know of and it also contains natural chelating acids that have the ability to aid with detoxification. Until recently though, rice bran fiber was viewed as useless because it rapidly became rancid and unusable, and it quickly lost its storehouse of nutrients. However, a new process has been developed which makes the oil fractions in rice bran fiber more chemically stable, so it can now be used in nutritional supplement formulas.

Research on fiber demonstrates that it supports the health of the colon and it promotes overall good health in general.[27] Strong evidence suggests that eating enough fiber helps to prevent atherosclerotic cardiovascular disease, and it decreases serum cholesterol and LDL cholesterol concentrations.[28] Fiber also lowers blood-glucose levels in diabetics. With regard to detoxification, it provides an internal cleansing and promotes healthy intestinal function. Fiber binds with toxic materials, helping to carry them out of the body, and it improves the ratio of toxic bacterial flora to friendly bacterial flora in the gut.

Fiber also protects us from the toxic substances that we produce ourselves. It not only lowers the absorption of carcinogens from our diet, it also reduces the conversion of bile salts released by the liver into potential carcinogens. We all produce toxic substances in our intestines—such as skatole, indole, and cadaverine—due to the incompletely digested protein substances in our body. These undigested proteins become highly toxic if they are not neutralized by adequate levels of antioxidants and fiber. For a healthy adult, the American Dietetic Association recommends a minimum of twenty to thirty-five grams of fiber per day.

D-Ribose

D-ribose (sometimes referred to as just ribose, although there are actually different forms of ribose) is a simple, naturally-occurring, five-carbon sugar that is found in all living cells. It's sweet to the taste, water-soluble, and critical to metabolism. D-ribose is used by the body to synthesize the universal energy molecule ATP (adenosine triphosphate), a nucleotide, produced by the mitochondria inside cells, that is responsible for the chemical energy that drives otherwise uphill biochemical reactions in the body. It is also used to make nucleic acids and the backbone of DNA and RNA molecules are composed of it.

DNA (deoxyribonucleic acid) is the long complex macromolecule—consisting of two interconnected helical strands—that resides in the nucleus of every living cell and encodes the genetic instructions for building each organism. RNA (ribonucleic acid) is the messenger molecule that encodes instructions from the DNA, and then transports these instructions outside the nucleus of the cell, where it puts them into action assembling proteins.

Research indicates that D-ribose supplements can help patients undergoing bypass surgery to recover more quickly.[29] Other studies have shown that D-ribose is good for cardiovascular health in general, and that it may have cardioprotective effects, particularly for the ischemic heart.[30] D-ribose has been shown to be effective in treating congestive heart failure and improving performance in athletes. It is also known to have anti-anxiety effects, without being sedating, and is sometimes used to control stress-related eating and drinking. Some people claim that D-ribose has antidepressant qualities as well.

By supplementing your diet with additional D-ribose you increase the rate at which ATP is generated, and this leads to an improvement in exercise performance and faster muscle growth. Supplemental D-ribose can increase the speed at which lost nucleotides are replaced and muscle fibers are repaired, and this is why there has been so much interest in the potential of D-ribose supplements to boost muscular performance in sports. D-ribose is important for detoxification because environmental toxins and heavy metals plug up many biochemical pathways and slow down many metabolic reactions in the body, resulting in lower energy. By replenishing our cells with an abundance of this simple sugar, we help to provide our bodies with the precursory material necessary for the metabolic reactions upon which life depends. This helps to restore the body's natural energy level and aids in the detoxification process.

Although it's essential for the biochemistry of life, D-ribose is not an essential nutrient. This means that it can be made in the body from other substances, such as glucose. However, we normally obtain D-ribose from our diet, because it's metabolically complex for the body to manufacture. Brewers yeast is a rich source of D-ribose. When D-ribose is taken as a nutritional supplement it bypasses the slow biochemical conversion steps needed by the body to normally create it and is readily available for the creation of more ATP. Research has shown that about three to five grams of ribose per day should provide enough in the bloodstream to ensure that the heart and skeletal-muscle cells have an adequate supply.

Saunas and Sweating

Another important way to help detoxify the body is by sweating from heat or exercise. The skin is the body's largest organ and it is one of the most important for detoxification. Sweating helps to remove mercury and other toxins from the body.[31] Saunas can be especially helpful as a way to induce sweating. There is an ancient tradition behind using temperature-raising methods to induce therapeutic sweating as a way of removing toxins. From the Roman Steam Bath to the Native American Sweat Lodge, people have been detoxifying themselves this way throughout human history.

There are a number of different types of saunas available. Some use conventional steam, some use heated rocks, and others use infrared heaters. There is some evidence that infrared saunas, which tend to be more comfortable than traditional saunas, may be the most efficient at detoxification. One study analyzed the chemical composition of sweat collected from people using hot rock saunas and compared it to the sweat collected from people using an infrared sauna. The hot rock sauna induced sweat contained more water and less toxins than the sweat induced by an infrared sauna. The hot rock sauna induced sweat was ninety-five to ninety-seven percent water, and the infrared sauna induced sweat was eighty to eighty-five percent water—the rest being composed of cholesterol, fat-soluble toxins, heavy metals, sulfuric acid, ammonia, sodium, and uric acid.

The temperature for a therapeutic sauna should be between a hundred forty to a hundred eighty degrees fahrenheit, in contrast to the two hundred to two hundred ten degrees fahrenheit temperature for a standard non-therapeutic sauna. It's important to shower and towel dry after a sauna because the removal of sweat prevents the reabsorption of toxins.

It's also important to drink adequate amounts of water while doing a sauna in order to avoid dehydration. It is suggested that one drink a minimum of two quarts of water before and after entering a sauna. It's also a good idea to replace the electrolytes that one loses to perspiration with grape or prune juice, and to drink vegetable juices (or take supplements) to replace the calcium and magnesium lost through the skin. Drinking plenty of water is an essential part of the detoxification process in general because more water helps to flush more toxins out of your body faster. It is suggested that one drink half of one's body weight—in ounces—of filtered or distilled water per day.

Drinking plenty of water, sweating, and taking herbal and nutritional supplements can dramatically help one's body to combat the vast armies of environmental toxins that invade it each day, but even the most effective techniques still leave a significant amount of heavy metals in our body. Sometimes these heavy metals will lie low and remain hidden in our bodies for years, only to resurface later, when our defenses are down and they can do greater harm.

Lead Stored in the Bones May Be Released During Menopause

Some of all those toxins and heavy metals that flood into our bodies cause havoc right away, while others that can't be eliminated are stored in fatty tissue and bone. In these parts of the body, heavy metals may be stored for years, being released during times of exercise, stress, or fasting.

In the Biosphere 2 project described previously, the environmental toxins that are stored in the fatty tissues of our bodies could be studied in an objective manner. Once the eight biospherians were sealed in their hermetically-sealed environment, no new toxins were introduced into their systems and they all lost weight. This set the stage for an ideal situation to study the toxins that are stored in our body fat. Roy Walford, the UCLA longevity researcher who participated in the project, took blood samples every day from the biospherians to measure the amount of toxins being released from their fatty tissue.

The results were not pretty. Not long after the project was underway, most of the biospherians had significant concentrations of DDT, DDE, and other highly toxic compounds that had not even been in use for years, circulating in their bloodstreams. These results were published in the journal *Toxicological Sciences* in 1999, showing that lipophilic compounds (those stored in fat) DDE and PCBs increased in the biospherians' blood as the they lost weight and then decreased as they put the weight back on after the two years.[32]

These stored toxins—that we all carry around in us—can be released into the circulatory system at a later time when the body is less equipped to deal effectively with them due to aging, illness, or an accident. This can be especially concerning for middle-aged women who are undergoing menopause, as elevated levels of lead have been found circulating in this portion of the population.[33]

It is known that bone mineral density decreases after menopause in women and that any lead that has been stored in the bones is then released into the body's circulatory system.[34] Some researchers have observed a significant increase in median blood lead levels associated with the bone mineral density decreases during menopause.[35]

A study done with more than two thousand women, between the ages of forty and fifty-nine, found that the quarter with the highest levels of lead in their blood were at 3.4 times the risk of developing high blood pressure than those with the lowest levels of lead.[36] This was despite the fact that these women had lower blood-lead levels than the U.S. government specifies as supposedly safe for adults. This evidence suggests that EDTA chelation therapy could be of benefit to women undergoing menopause as it binds to the circulating lead and eliminates it from the body.

The combined evidence from over forty years of chelation therapy research suggests that EDTA may be the most powerful tool that we have available for detoxifying our bodies from lead and the other dangerous heavy metals that threaten our health and well-being with every breath that we take.

How Does EDTA Work?

Chelation is a natural chemical process that goes on continually in our bodies. The transportation and migration of zinc and iron in and out of cells are achieved by a chelating process, and the iron in hemoglobin is a chelated metal. The most abundant chelator in the body is a substance called albumen and higher levels of it have been associated with a longer lifespan. Metals and minerals are continuously binding and recombining with other substances in the human body and EDTA utilizes this natural process to our advantage.

A chelating agent has a binding capacity that can be mathematically determined. EDTA, for instance, has at least six pairs of unshared electrons that can bind to atoms or groups of atoms carrying a positive charge. Here's how it works. The disodium-salt portion of the EDTA molecule has a weaker molecular bond than do the metals or minerals that it chelates. As the minerals or metals bind with the EDTA, the weak disodium-salt bond is replaced with a new and stronger bond to the metal or mineral. This process then begins to neutralize the metal or mineral's toxic properties and prepares it for elimination from the body. The chelation process all happens relatively quickly, as the biologic half-life of EDTA, after intravenous administration, is approximately one hour.

EDTA's only action in the body is to alter the distribution of metals and minerals. It enters and exits the body very quickly and is never metabolized. In less than an hour after an intravenous infusion of EDTA, half of it has already been excreted in the urine—unchanged except for the metal ions and minerals that have binded to it during its journey through the circulatory system. It is due to this ability that EDTA initially attracted the attention of physicians and medical researchers. For people who accidentally exposed themselves to large doses of toxic heavy metals, like lead, EDTA worked like magic and its efficacy as a remover of metal ions from the body is relied upon in modern medicine for treating heavy metal toxicity.

Besides removing heavy metals from the body, EDTA also alters and reshuffles the distribution of metals and minerals in the body, and this may play a role in some of EDTA's unexplained health benefits. The EDTA molecule is not altered or degraded in any way as it travels through the body and it never enters into metabolic pathways. All that EDTA does is attract metal ions that bind to it. However, sometimes after EDTA binds with a specific metal ion it later encounters another metal ion that it has an even stronger affinity with. In these instances the original metal ion is then dropped and the newly encountered metal ion is substituted in its place. In this way a redistribution of the metals and minerals in the body may occur without necessarily removing them all, and this may play a role in EDTA's clinical benefits.

While it is well-known that minute amounts of heavy metals can have severe physiological or neurological effects, few people are aware that even essential elements have the potential to be toxic in excess. Dr. Frustaci and his colleagues in Italy have published data demonstrating that essential trace elements accumulate to potentially toxic levels in diseased tissues. When the young and healthy myocardial cells from control subjects are compared with the diseased cells of ischemic myocardium patients we see a significant accumulation of essential trace elements. These trace elements can reach extremely high levels. For example, zinc increases by two hundred eighty percent, chromium increases by five hundred twenty percent, and iron increases by four hundred percent. It's important to point out that there is only a narrow margin between normal and toxic levels of these metallic trace elements. Just three or four times the normal amount of these trace elements can poison cellular metabolism.

Because toxic metals also increase in diseased tissue—but less so than the essential elements—it appears that EDTA chelation therapy may be bestowing some of its health benefits by restoring a more normal distribution of essential metallic elements within the body. Some researchers believe that this action may actually be as important— possibly even more important—than the enhanced excretion of toxic metals. However, although it remains unclear at this point exactly how important this reshuffling of essential trace elements is as a mechanism of action in chelation therapy, we know that removing toxic heavy metals from the body can only be a good thing because their presence in our bodies unquestionably poisons cellular metabolism.

How Does EDTA Affect Bone Density Levels?

Since EDTA binds to calcium there was initially some concern that chelation therapy could be robbing people's bodies of needed calcium. If this were true it would be especially concerning for people who are vulnerable to bone density loss, such as osteoporosis patients. However studies have verified that there is no decrease in people's bone density levels following EDTA chelation therapy and that the therapy does not cause calcium depletion of the bones.[37]

In fact, in those patients who had some degree of osteoporosis there was a slight but statistically significant improvement in bone density readings. In other words, EDTA actually stimulated a regrowth of the bone in those patients affected with osteoporosis. Researchers concluded that their results indicate that EDTA therapy might be beneficial to bone growth in some cases. So, although EDTA chelation therapy has been shown to reduce calcium accumulation in the blood vessels, it is actually used as a treatment for osteoporosis because it has been shown to stimulate bone growth and to make bones stronger.

How does this work? According to Dr. Gordon, "Disodium EDTA actually stimulates bone growth because it ties up the calcium that's in the blood. When this happens the body thinks that there's a shortage of calcium, and it turns on the parathyroid hormone. The parathyroid hormone then mobilizes that calcium that has been building up in your artery. We can lower that content of calcium in your vascular tissue, and, amazingly enough, that same parathyroid hormone switch will make you turn on bone growth again. It's a very exciting process."

EDTA Effectively Removes Heavy Metals from the Body

We know that EDTA chelation therapy can effectively remove heavy metals from the body and we know that it can promote a multitude of health benefits. Although we don't know exactly why many of these health benefits occur, the evidence is beginning to look more and more like it supports the notion that the majority of health benefits attributed to chelation therapy can be adequately explained by heavy metal detoxification. For example, urine and fecal analysis confirm that a substantial amount of toxic heavy metals are being removed from the body during EDTA chelation therapy and this generally correlates with the measured and reported increase in health benefits.

The improved circulation and cardiovascular function that many people experience as a result of chelation therapy, in most cases, has nothing to do with arterial plaque removal, and it appears to be the result of treating endothelial dysfunction. The endothelium is a layer of thin specialized cells that line the interior surface of blood vessels throughout the entire circulatory system—from the heart muscle to the smallest capillary. By lowering lead levels in the endothelium EDTA chelation therapy improves nitric oxide production, which is essential for proper cardiovascular health.

Since the reduction of blood, oxygen, and nutrients due to poor circulation is linked to almost all major diseases, chelation therapy can be used to effectively treat many health conditions—including some conditions that medical science currently has no other effective treatments for, like aging. In the next chapter we'll look at how EDTA chelation therapy affects circulation, nitric oxide production, and cardiovascular health.

Chapter 3

BLOOD CIRCULATION AND CARDIOVASCULAR HEALTH

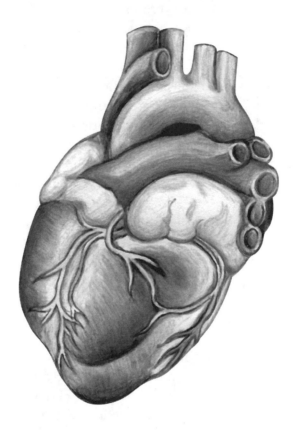

EDTA chelation therapy does far more than just remove dangerous heavy metals from the body. Numerous scientific studies have demonstrated EDTA chelation therapy's efficacy in treating cardiovascular disease and improving cardiovascular health.[1,2,3,4] In fact, the first reports of improved cardiovascular health began to roll in only shortly after physicians began utilizing EDTA's ability to remove lead from the body. Today, studies show that EDTA chelation therapy does much better than bypass surgery, angioplasty, or medications as a primary treatment for most cardiovascular disease.[5,6]

Early studies conducted by Norman Clarke at the Providence Hospital in Detroit, Michigan, in 1955, found that EDTA dissolves unwanted calcium deposits called "metastatic calcium," and that it can be effective in removing these calcium deposits from the body.[7] In the first systematic study of EDTA—which was published a year later—twenty patients with confirmed heart disease were given a series of thirty intravenous EDTA treatments. Nineteen of the patients experienced improvement, as measured by an increase in physical activity.[8]

Dr. Clarke's 1956 study showed significant improvements in patients suffering from angina pectoris after being treated with EDTA. The patients reported a consistent decrease or disappearance in anginal symptoms, and, in some cases, there was a disappearance of abnormalities in electrocardiograms that had been present for the two years preceding the onset of EDTA therapy. Then, in 1960, another study found that three months of EDTA treatments caused a decrease in the severity and frequency of anginal episodes, increased work capacity, improved electrocardiogram results, and significantly reduced the use of the anti-angina drug nitroglycerin.[9]

A retrospective study conducted by Drs. Hancke and Flytlie in 1993 followed four hundred seventy patients with cardiovascular disease who received intravenous EDTA chelation therapy.[11] The results showed significant improvements for eighty to ninety-one percent of the patients. Ninety-two patients in the study had been referred for surgical procedures, but after receiving intravenous EDTA chelation therapy, only ten still needed surgery. Avoiding surgery saved an estimated three million dollars in surgical and hospital fees, as well as a lengthy recovery period. Drs. Hancke and Flytlie concluded that EDTA therapy is "safe, effective, and results in cost savings."

Another study conducted by Richard Casdorph in the late 90s demonstrated EDTA chelation therapy's efficacy in treating arteriosclerotic heart disease.[12] Patients with arteriosclerotic heart disease were studied before and after the intravenous administration of EDTA chelation therapy, and a significant improvement in cardiovascular function was reported, as evidenced by a measurement of the left ventricular "ejection fraction." The "ejection fraction" is the amount of blood pumped out of a ventricle with each heart beat, which is used as a measurement of the heart's efficiency. In Casdorph's study, the resting ejection fraction was measured in patients before and after EDTA chelation therapy, and a significant improvement in the left ventricular ejection fraction was reported after the treatment. The results demonstrated that all eighteen patients in the study improved clinically, and in all but two of the patients there was a complete subsidence of angina during the course of EDTA chelation therapy.

Some of the best evidence supporting EDTA chelation therapy's efficacy in treating cardiovascular disease comes from a meta-analysis done by Terry Chappell and John Stahl.[13] A meta-analysis is a study that combines the results from many previously published studies so that they can all be evaluated statistically as a single study. Drs. Chappell and Stahl combined the results from nineteen studies that evaluated EDTA chelation therapy's ability to improve cardiovascular function, with data from 22,765 patients. The meta-analysis revealed a correlation coefficient of 0.88, which indicates a high positive relationship between EDTA therapy and improved cardiovascular function. Eighty-seven percent of the patients included in the meta-analysis demonstrated clinical improvement by objective testing.

Another meta-analysis done by Drs. Chappell and Stahl combined the reported results from previously unpublished "file drawer" data from thirty-two clinicians who utilize EDTA chelation therapy in their practice, so as to address the concern of skeptics who pointed out that physicians might only be reporting positive data in the literature.[14] Objective measurements demonstrated an improvement in cardio-vascular health in eighty-eight percent of the 1,241 patients studied, which is essentially the same as the results from the meta-analysis of published data. In other words, the data supporting the claim that EDTA chelation therapy improves cardiovascular health is quite substantial and has been replicated many times.

However, the primary criticism of EDTA chelation therapy is that its cardiovascular benefits remain unproven because large-scale, randomized, double-blind controlled studies have not been conducted. The reason why this hasn't been done yet is because funding such a study costs many millions of dollars and the pharmaceutical companies—who normally fund studies on this scale—have nothing to gain from it because the patent on EDTA expired in 1969. Nonetheless, the first large-scale, randomized, double-blind controlled study is right now being conducted by the U.S. government. Currently, the National Institutes of Health has a five year study underway, involving 2,372 participants, called the Trial to Access Chelation Therapy or TACT study, that began in August of 2002. This is the first large-scale study looking at whether EDTA chelation therapy is "safe and effective for people with coronary heart disease," and although twenty-nine million dollars is being spent on the study some chelation-practicing physicians have strong criticisms of this work.

According to Dr. Gordon, "The TACT study is designed to merely test one thing—will people who use some chelation with an oral vitamin and mineral supplement during those five years have less heart attacks, or less of need for surgery, than the people who got a placebo? This study is not near and dear to me because it's using the old outdated sodium EDTA that requires four hour treatments, which nobody really has time for anymore. The study really came out of my incorrect belief thirty years ago that I had found the magic bullet to clean everybody's arteries, and we now know that we don't have it. So, since I'm really much more focused on the long-term implications today, I'm sorry to see us waste our money on a study that only does a few chelations and then follows subjects for a few years. It will probably come out as a slight benefit but nowhere near the kind of benefit that one is able to achieve if people are put on to the oral chelation after the I.V.s."

What Causes Cardiovascular Disease?

Heart disease is the number one leading cause of death for both women and men in the United States. According to the American Heart Association, more than 910,000 Americans die of heart disease a year, and more than seventy million Americans live with some form of cardiovascular disease—such as high blood pressure, congenital heart defects, angina, or the aftereffects from a stroke or heart attack. Worldwide, coronary heart disease (the principal type of heart disease) kills more than seven million people each year.

The most common form of cardiovascular disease is coronary artery disease (CAD). Approximately seven million Americans suffer from

CAD. It is the leading cause of death among Americans; more than five hundred thousand Americans die of CAD-related heart attacks each year. In CAD the coronary arteries—the vessels that bring oxygen-rich blood to the tissues of the heart—become blocked by deposits of a fatty substance called plaque.

As this fatty substance builds up in the arteries, they become narrower and narrower. This means that less oxygen and nutrients are able to reach the heart. This condition can lead to serious medical conditions, such as angina—pain caused by not enough oxygen-rich blood reaching the heart—as well as heart attacks and strokes. However, a person with CAD may or may not have symptoms. Symptoms may include chest pain from angina, shortness of breath, nausea, light-headedness, or cold sweats—but a lack of symptoms doesn't necessary imply cardiovascular health.

There are different types of plaque that can potentially clog our circulatory systems. For many years it was thought that the large calcified plaque deposits growing on the walls of arteries and veins, which obstruct the flow of blood through the circulatory system, were the leading cause of heart attacks and strokes. We now know that this isn't the case. It isn't the hard plaque deposits in our circulatory system that are so dangerous, but rather the soft, relatively small plaque deposits that form within our vessel walls—which can easily rupture because they are so vulnerable—that present the greatest risk, as they can cause blood vessels to become completely blocked.

Large, calcified plaque deposits are actually relatively stable. These deposits have a hard calcified covering on them and because of this they are less likely to crack. The less stable and more dynamic soft plaque deposits are much more likely to suddenly crack off or rupture. If this happens, then the body immediately forms a clot to try to heal the rupture, and this may result in a total blockage of blood flow. When the blood supply reaching the heart gets cut off sufficiently a heart attack (or myocardial infarction) occurs. When this happens the supply of oxygen reaching the heart becomes so poor that part of the heart muscle dies. If a sufficiently large portion of the heart is affected, then it may no longer be able to pump blood efficiently to the rest of the body, resulting in death or chronic heart failure.

What Can Be Done To Reduce the Formation of Soft Plaque Deposits?

Soft plaque deposits hide inside the walls of our blood vessels and their usually silent and invisible presence presents one of the greatest dangers to our cardiovascular health. In many cases the deposits cause no obvious blockage, or loss of blood flow, until the often-fatal rupture.

The good news is that soft plaque deposits are more easily reversible than hard plaque deposits. Levels of the two types of plaque are related to one another, since the same process appears to result in both forms. One prevalent theory on the origin of hard plaque deposits is that they result from the body's attempt to protect the vessel walls from vulnerable plaque deposits by covering them with a hard, calcified coating. This theory helps to explain why bypass surgery and balloon angioplasty don't slow down the process of soft or hard plaque formation, as it appears that cardiovascular disease isn't localized in any one area and is present in the entire circulatory system. In fact, we now know that these surgical procedures often actually increase plaque deposit formation and accelerate the development of cardiovascular disease.

A study conducted in 1999 by David Waters at the University of California dramatically shifted our understanding in this area.[15] In the study, Waters randomly assigned patients who had been referred for angioplasty surgery into two groups. One group received the surgery and the standard follow-up care. The other group received cholesterol-lowering statin drugs but no surgery. The non-surgery group actually had fewer heart attacks and fewer visits to the hospital for chest pain than the surgery group. This new understanding of the difference between soft plaque and hard plaque helps to explain why bypass and angioplasty surgeries don't usually help much and can actually make matters worse. It also helps to explain why heart attacks typically strike with no apparent warning, and often to people who seem to be healthy, according to conventional diagnostic methods.

Most physicians and medical researchers believe that soft plaque formation and other forms of cardiovascular disease are caused by a combination of genetic and environmental factors. One of the best predictors of whether or not someone will get cardiovascular disease is whether or not his or her parents had it. Diet and exercise are thought to play major roles in cardiovascular health. Many physicians encourage people to eat low fat, low-cholesterol diets, and to exercise regularly, as a link between cholesterol, saturated fats, physical inactivity, and heart disease have been found. High blood pressure, high cholesterol levels, a sedentary lifestyle, and increasing age are all known to be contributing factors in the development of cardiovascular disease.

Dietary experts tell us that the primary fats to avoid are saturated animal fats (found in meat and dairy products) and trans fats (or hydrogenated vegetable oils). But certain types of fat are absolutely essential for proper health. These fats are called essential fatty acids, and they are vital for good cardiovascular health. Unfortunately, the average American diet usually contains high levels of the dangerous forms of fat and low levels of the beneficial types of heart-healthy fat. The Omega-3, Omega-6, and Omega-9 essential fatty acids necessary for cardiovascular health can be found in fish oil, hemp seed oil, and flax seeds. Some other important nutrients that have been shown to improve cardiovascular health are vitamin E (mixed tocopherols and tocotrienols), vitamin C, and coenzyme Q-10.

Coenzyme Q10 (CoQ10) has been shown to be particularly important for cardiovascular health. This fat-soluble, vitamin-like substance plays a critical role in the mitochondria's production of ATP by shuttling electrons back and forth between enzymes. Many thousands of scientific studies have been done on CoQ10, demonstrating its many benefits on cardiovascular health, and that it is often deficient among patients with cardiovascular disease. CoQ10 is a powerful antioxidant that has been shown to improve all known forms of cardiovascular disease. Taking CoQ10 supplements is especially important for people taking statin drugs, as these drugs interfere with one's ability to synthesize CoQ10, causing one to have lower levels as a result.

Regular exercise is important for cardiovascular health. A diet rich in fresh organic vegetables, that is low in saturated animal fat, trans fat, refined sugar, and carbohydrates, has been shown to reduce the risk of heart disease. Omega-3 fatty acids, CoQ10, and vitamins C and E have all been shown to be essential for cardiovascular health. But that's only the tip of the iceberg with regard to what we can do to insure our cardiovascular vitality. As we've learned, EDTA chelation therapy can also dramatically improve cardiovascular health and significantly improve circulation. In fact, it sets the gold standard for how to insure vibrant and radiant cardiovascular health—but how does it work?

How Does EDTA Improve Cardiovascular Health?

The reported cardiovascular improvements in the studies discussed above have generally been attributed to the removal of metastatic calcification from the arterial wall or to EDTA's interference with slow calcium currents. Some researchers believe that EDTA improves cardiovascular health by blocking the slow calcium currents in the arterial wall (that are responsible for the electrical activation and contraction of smooth muscle cells), and that this results in arterial vasodilatation, similar to the way that calcium channel blocking drugs work.

EDTA binds to calcium in much the same way as it does to heavy metals, and this can help to remove unwanted calcium deposits from the body. Because EDTA dissolves metastatic calcification and improves cardiovascular health, it was thought that EDTA removed hard calcified plaque deposits from the arterial walls. For many years chelation therapy-practicing-physicians believed that EDTA worked by "clawing" away those hard calcium deposits in people's arteries and veins, or by dissolving away the calcified blockages like a biological version of Drano® or Roto-Rooter®.

However, we now know that this assumption doesn't hold up in scientific tests, as studies have failed to confirm that EDTA removes calcium deposits from the arterial walls to any significant degree.[16] Even though EDTA dissolves metastatic calcium and improves blood circulation, studies show that it appears to have little effect on cardiovascular blockages—at least not to the extent that would explain the benefits that it generates. Nonetheless, people who use EDTA continue to show improved circulation and other fairly dramatic cardiovascular benefits.[17]

So if EDTA isn't clearing calcified plaque deposits out of the vascular system then how is it improving cardiovascular health? Currently, no one knows for sure what the answer to this question is, but the cardiovascular improvements are undeniable. At present, the mechanism by which these benefits occur remains unknown, although some compelling evidence suggests that understanding a substance in the body called nitric oxide may help us to solve the mystery.

The Importance of Nitric Oxide

Nitric oxide (NO)—a gas composed of nitrogen and oxygen—plays an important role in the body's biochemistry. (NO should not be confused with nitrous oxide, N20, the analgesic gas that makes you giggle at the dentist's office.) Also known as "endothelium-derived relaxing factor," NO is a key biological messenger, playing a role in a variety of biochemical processes. It is essential for everything from proper cardiovascular health to firm penile erections, and it appears to control a limitless range of functions in the body. NO helps to control blood circulation, blood vessel dilatation, neurotransmission, modulation of the hair cycle, and it regulates activities of the brain, lungs, liver, kidneys, stomach, gut, genitals, and other organs.

NO controls the action of virtually every orifice in the body, from swallowing to defecating. The immune system uses NO to help fight infections—viral, bacterial and parasitic—as well as tumors. It is a mediator in inflammation and rheumatism. NO also acts as a neurotransmitter in the brain, communicating messages between brain cells, where it is associated with the learning process, memory, sleeping, and pain perception. It regulates blood pressure, and it causes penile erections by dilating blood vessels. Viagra's phenomenal success is due to the drug's ability to enhance the effects of NO.

NO is synthesized from arginine and oxygen by substances called "nitric oxide synthases," enzymes, and by a sequential reduction of inorganic nitrate. The endothelium (inner lining) of blood vessels use nitric oxide to signal the surrounding smooth muscle to relax, thus dilating the artery and increasing blood flow. The production of nitric oxide has been noted to increase in high-altitude populations for this affect, which helps people to avoid becoming oxygen deficient in thin air.

NO is essential for healthy cardiovascular function. The heart medication nitroglycerin—which is used to treat angina pectoris—works because it is quickly converted by the body into NO, where it acts as a vasodilator. It appears that EDTA chelation therapy operates in a similar fashion, only more gradually. Although EDTA isn't converted into NO, like nitroglycerin it also increases NO levels in the body and it enhances vasodilatation.[18] How does EDTA accomplish this?

According to Dr. Gordon, "The mechanism by which EDTA effects nitric oxide levels has to do with the levels of lead that accumulate in all of our tissues, and everyone today is toxic with lead. If you look at the Periodic Table of Elements you will see that the atomic structure of lead and zinc are directly related to each other. When you realize how much lead we have in our bodies you begin to see the problem. As we raise the levels of lead we are actually plugging lead into key enzyme functions in our body that normally zinc would have fulfilled.[19] Some of those enzymes are called nitric oxide syntheses. These are the key enzymes that are responsible for this job of attempting to help our body keep a healthy balance of blood flow by making nitric oxide out of the arginine and related amino acids that we get in our diet. If you can make good levels of nitric oxide, then you're going to have your blood vessels relaxed instead of constricted. If they're relaxed, then they're open and they let more blood go through. The net result is that the person then has less angina and more ability to walk miles without getting leg cramps."

As we learned in the last chapter, every person on this planet is suffering from some degree of heavy metal poisoning. We all have too much lead in our body, and when it's there it is adversely effecting the tissue that it accumulates in. So if your heart has too much lead in it then the pumping function of your heart will be affected. In fact, there's a disease called "idiopathic dilated hypertrophic cardiomyopathy," where the heart muscle is enlarged, and when the tissue is analyzed it can have as much as a ten thousand-fold increase in the levels of mercury, lead, or cadmium.

Having toxic metals like lead, cadmium, and mercury in the heart muscle lowers its efficiency and puts people at risk for heart disease, but heavy metals affect more than just the heart—they affect the entire cardiovascular system. Blood flow through the capillaries, arteries and veins is affected by the level of heavy metals in the body. For example, when lead levels go up and the body is no longer able to convert the amino acid arginine into NO, the circulatory system as a whole becomes less relaxed and more constricted. Using EDTA chelation therapy to clear away the heavy metals helps the body to produce NO, which dilates and relaxes the circulatory system. This appears to be one of the primary reasons why EDTA chelation improves cardiovascular health, but there are more.

The Importance of Reducing Inflammation

Inflammation is a characteristic reaction of tissues to injury or disease that is marked by swelling, redness, heat, and usually pain. However, there is also a common form of inflammation known as 'silent inflammation' that is painless but extremely dangerous. Silent inflammation, which is often linked to diet, has been correlated with a higher incidence of cardiovascular disease and has been identified as one of the most important factors in the formation of plaque and arterial disease.

Silent inflammation is caused by elevated insulin levels in the body, which are caused by too much refined sugar and too many simple carbohydrates in one's diet. Many people are unaware of the fact that reducing sugars and carbohydrates in one's diet is every bit as important as cutting out the wrong types of fat, if one is interested in maintaining cardiovascular health as he or she ages. Carbohydrates are converted by the body into sugars, which elevates blood-glucose levels. In response to the elevated levels of sugar, the pancreas releases insulin into the bloodstream, which allows cells to metabolize the sugar and helps the body to compound the storage of fat. Too much fat storage can be a problem because obesity is linked to silent inflammation and cardiovascular disease.

So the more sugar and carbohydrates that one has with a meal, the higher one's insulin levels rise as a result, the more fat one gains, and the greater one's problem with silent inflammation becomes. Insulin also stimulates the production of enzymes that make the building blocks of substances called "inflammatory eicosanoids," which are hormones that travel between cells and cause inflammation. This elevation in insulin levels, and the increase in fat storage and inflammation that results, are some of the primary reasons why obesity is linked to cardiovascular disease. The more obese you are, the more insulin you're making, and the more inflammation you're generating—which leads to plaque formation and arterial disease.

This is why having a low-glycemic, anti-inflammatory diet is so important. Fish oil supplements, mentioned above as being an important dietary source of essential fatty acids, have also been shown to reduce inflammation, as well as the risk of a sudden-death heart attack by fifty to eighty percent, depending on the dose. The primary benefits from fish oil come from the long-chain fatty acids—such as EPA and DHA— which, at high enough levels, have profound anti-inflammatory effects. Even as little as two meals per week of fatty cold water fish could give you a forty to fifty percent reduction in your risk of sudden-death heart attacks. However, the best way to get your fish oil is from a highly purified, highly refined source that concentrates the important essential fatty acids and removes the dangerous toxins and heavy metals.

EDTA chelation therapy is also thought to reduce inflammation, due to its powerful antioxidant properties (which will be discussed in chapter 5), as one of the ways that it improves cardiovascular health. EDTA chelation therapy may partially work by reducing the damaging effects of oxidative stress on the walls of the blood vessels, and this could reduce inflammation in the arteries and improve blood vessel function. Reducing inflammation is extremely important for maintaining cardiovascular health, but there are still other ways that EDTA chelation therapy can help us to keep our hearts and circulatory systems healthy.

Is Heart Disease Caused by an Infectious Pathogen?

There is a growing body of evidence, and a compelling theoretical foundation, to support the notion that much of cardiovascular disease might actually be caused by an infectious pathogen, such as a virus or a form of bacteria.[20] Some evolutionary biologists are making a strong case for the idea that many of the supposedly benign microbes that chronically infect our bodies may not be quite as benign as has been previously thought.

Conventional wisdom tells us that cardiovascular disease is generally caused by a combination of genetic and environmental factors, such as diet and exercise, while ignoring the possibility that it may be largely caused by slow-acting, chronically-infecting pathogens that don't have acute phases of harm. Paul Ewald—who is at the forefront of the biologists championing this idea—says that our focus in medicine on acute infections that require immediate attention has blinded us from seeing the long-term dangers of chronic infections.

For example, it wasn't until 1982 that we discovered that most cases of cervical cancer are actually caused by certain strains of the human papilloma virus. Ewald believes that many of the chronic diseases that plague the human species—such as heart disease and different forms of cancer—will eventually reveal themselves as being caused by similar, seemingly benign, slow-acting pathogens that build up substantial damage over time. In chapter 5, where we discuss disease prevention, this theory, and the evidence supporting it, will be explained in greater detail. However, because of EDTA's antiviral properties, it's important to point out that this may be yet another mode of action in EDTA's ability to improve cardiovascular health. There is still one more.

EDTA's Anti-clotting Properties

More than a third of Americans die of a heart attacks or stroke, most of which are caused by a blood clot. Medical experts are pretty much in agreement today that well over eighty percent of heart attacks are, in fact, actually due to a blood clot. This is why so many people take aspirin, which has been found to lower the incidence of heart attacks and strokes due to its blood thinning abilities and anti-inflammatory properties.[21] However, aspirin only prevents one type of blood-clotting—what is called platelet aggregation—and this is only a small portion of what's necessary to prevent cardiovascular disease. Aspirin doesn't effect the coagulation of blood.

Many people rely on aspirin for protection from cardiovascular disease, however studies show that thirty percent of people experience no benefit from aspirin—in terms of blood-clotting prevention—and aspirin use is not without its own risks.[22] Over three thousand people die each year from ingesting aspirin. The very same anti-clotting effect that helps to prevent heart attacks and clot-caused strokes raises the risk of bleeding problems, such as hemorrhagic strokes (strokes due to bleeding) and gastrointestinal bleeding from ulcers. EDTA's anti-clotting properties, on the other hand, work synergistically with the systems in the body and there aren't any serious risks associated with its use.

The body's natural anti-clotting, anticoagulant factor is a substance called heparin. Heparin is a natural part of the body's blood-clotting control system and it is used to prevent clots. If you have a blood clot clogging your circulatory system—as in the case of a stroke—physicians can use heparin to treat it. Unfortunately, we normally don't have enough heparin in our circulatory system to handle the acute situation when a heart attack or stroke is occurring. In fact, there is evidence that heparin activity deficiency may be an important factor in atherogenesis. People are taught to rush to the hospital to get a heparin-like treatment known as a "tissue plasmagin activator," which can dissolve a clot. But it may be wiser to try to prevent the clot from occurring in the first place.

EDTA chelation therapy has been shown to favorably influence the hypercoagulability of blood in the circulatory system and to reduce the incidence of blood-clotting.[23] These effects can be significantly boosted by combining EDTA with other substances that give it a heparin-like effect. My coauthor's own work has been in the area of developing formulas to help prevent blood clots using EDTA in conjunction with biochemical derivatives from valuable marine plants. Research by Lester Morrison—when he was the head of the Institute of Atereosclerosois Research at Loma Linda—provided the groundwork for development in this area. Dr. Morrison found that certain kinds of seaweed substances called mucopolysaccharides—like carrageenan, which are found in red algae—can help prevent blood clots.

However, Dr. Morrison's research only studied how carrageenans effect blood-clotting on their own, and he was having to use large quantities of the fiber-like substance—almost a third of a glass—in order to get all of the benefits. Dr. Gordon and colleagues found that orally administered EDTA works synergistically with carrageenan to help prevent blood clots, and that these two substances work far more efficiently together than each on their own. This combination has been shown to offer significant protection from blood clotting, without the serious dangers associated with anti-clotting pharmaceutical drugs.

EDTA chelation therapy is an invaluable tool for preventing cardiovascular disease, and it becomes far more powerful when it is combined with carrageenans, and the nutritional supplements discussed in this chapter and the previous chapter. Having a healthy cardiovascular system adequately nourishes all the organs and tissues, bathing them in nutrients and allowing the other systems in the body to function more efficiently. A strong heart makes for a strong mind. In the next chapter we'll be looking at how EDTA chelation therapy effects autism, cognition, and mental health.

Chapter 4

EDTA AND MENTAL HEALTH

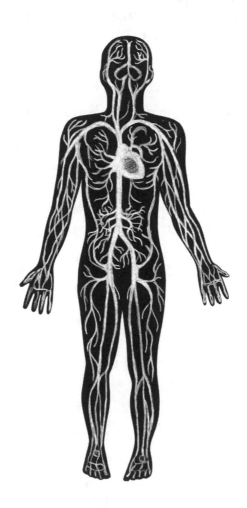

Because EDTA chelation therapy increases circulation to the brain, it can also help to improve cognitive function and memory. Chelation therapy removes aluminum from the body—which has been incriminated in senile and pre-senile dementia—as well as other toxic heavy metals which are known to cause brain damage.[1] Because of these properties, it has been shown to provide benefits in the treatment of autism, senile dementia, and Alzheimer's disease.[2]

Many people also report antidepressant and psycho-energizing effects from using EDTA. Additionally, it appears that healthy people with good brain functioning can also benefit from the cognitive-enhancing, memory-boosting, and mind-clarifying properties of EDTA. In other words, in addition to making us stronger and healthier, it appears that EDTA chelation therapy can also make us smarter and happier.

Brain Science 101

The adult human brain—which generally weighs around three pounds and is approximately the size of a large grapefruit—is the most complexly organized matter that we know of in the universe. It is composed of approximately a hundred billion neurons (brain cells), which are densely interconnected with one another. Each neuron generally connects to tens of thousands of other neurons and there are over a million billion interconnections between neurons in the brain.

Neurons are cells with branching root-like structures called dendrites and a single thin neuronal branch called an axon. They communicate with one another using these branching, interconnected structures. Neurons use dendrites to receive chemical or electrical signals from other neurons and they use their axon to transmit chemical or electrical signals to other neurons. Axons and dendrites are separated from one another by an extremely small gap called a synapse. It is in that tiny space that neurons send electrical impulses, and chemical messengers called neurotransmitters, to one another. This triggers effects in other neurons, and these electrochemical reactions ultimately encode for how we perceive the world and remember what we experience. Physical sensations, sensory perceptions, emotions, and thoughts are all created through the brain's (largely mysterious) electrochemical language.

The human brain sits majestically on top of the central nervous system, like a queen on her throne, and is intimately connected to every other system in the body. The relationship between the mind and the body, as it relates to medicine, is too big of a topic for this book, however, it is important to point out that studies by neuroscience researcher Candace Pert and others have demonstrated that the mind and body operate as parts of a single integrated system. The placebo effect—simply believing that a treatment will help—is one of the most powerful effects that we know of in medicine, and simply having a positive optimistic attitude toward life has been shown to have major health benefits. Mind-body medicine is discussed at length in my previous book, *Mavericks of Medicine* (Smart Publications, 2006).

Brain disorders are the most disturbing, intriguing, and perplexing of all medical disorders because they effect the very nature of who we are and how we perceive the world. Because the brain is so complex, when something goes wrong, treating it has proven to be a serious challenge. Therefore, any possibly overlooked treatment that has been shown to have efficiency in this area should be viewed with an open mind. But first, let's take a look at the most common form of all brain disorders—cerebrovascular disease.

What Causes Cerebrovascular Disease?

Cerebrovascular disease is caused by damaged blood vessels in the brain, which results in reduced blood flow, and sometimes manifests as a stroke. Strokes are the third leading cause of death in the U.S. and they are the number one cause of serious long-term disability. A stroke occurs when blood flow to the brain is interrupted—due to a vascular blockage or hemorrhage—significantly long enough for a population of neurons in the brain to die from a lack of oxygen and nutrients. Strokes that aren't fatal may lead to permanent paralysis, memory loss, personality changes, and other serious neurological or psychological problems.

The damaged blood vessels in the brain can become blocked because of fatty plaque deposits, or a wandering blood clot, and this can prevent the flow of blood from reaching certain parts of the brain. About eighty percent of strokes are caused by a blocked blood vessel. Sometimes the blood vessels may also leak, break, or burst—spewing blood into the surrounding brain tissue—resulting in a hemorrhagic stroke. This accounts for the other twenty percent of strokes. People with diabetes and presenile Alzheimer's disease are at higher risk of stroke and other forms of cerebrovascular disease.

If someone appears to be having a stroke, treatment is required immediately and every single second counts. The five major warning signs of a stroke are: (1) a sudden numbness or weakness in the muscles of the face, arms, or legs, especially on one side of the body; (2) a sudden feeling of confusion, or trouble speaking or understanding what people are saying; (3) sudden trouble seeing in one or both eyes; (4) sudden trouble walking, feelings of dizziness, or a loss of coordination; and (5) a severe, sudden headache with no obvious cause.

A simple way for people who are not trained as health professionals to recognize if someone has just had a stroke is by asking the person to do three simple things: smile, speak, and raise both arms. If the person is manifesting any of the symptoms discussed above, or has difficulty performing any of these simple actions, one should immediately call 911 and seek emergency medical treatment.

The most common form of cerebrovascular disease is due to atherosclerosis (or narrowing) of the blood vessels within the brain, as a result of plaque deposits. There may also be a defect or weakness in a blood vessel in the brain which can cause an aneurysm (ballooning of an artery). Both of these conditions make it more likely that a stroke will occur, and both can be helped through the use of EDTA chelation therapy.

EDTA Chelation Therapy's Efficacy in Treating Brain Disorders

Researchers have demonstrated that EDTA chelation therapy may have efficacy in treating brain disorders caused by poor circulation or the accumulation of toxic heavy metals. A study conducted by H. Richard Casdorph demonstrated that EDTA chelation therapy can significantly improve cerebral blood flow.[3] Fifteen patients with well-documented cerebral blood flow impairment were studied. All fifteen patients improved clinically following the EDTA chelation therapy treatments, including one patient who showed little or no measurable improvement in blood flow.

Studies have shown increased concentrations of aluminum in the brains of patients with Alzheimer's disease.[4,5] No offense meant to those who appreciate 'heavy metal' music, but being a 'metal head' may be something that you want to avoid—at least in the literal sense—as heavy metals are known to cause brain damage. Studies by the National Center for Environmental Health and Center for Disease Control studies show a correlation between lower lead levels and a higher I.Q., as well as correlations with lower lead levels and increased worker productivity.[6]

Since EDTA binds to aluminum and is known to carry it out of the body, it makes sense that EDTA chelation therapy may be helpful in preventing or treating Alzheimer's disease and other brain disorders. Although there haven't been any studies performed yet in this area, preliminary results reported by H. Richard Casdorph indicate that some forms of Alzheimer's disease appear to respond to chelation therapy, at least in the early stages.[7] EDTA chelation therapy has also been found to be especially effective in treating autistic children.

What is Autism?

Autism is a largely mysterious neurodevelopmental disorder that usually manifests in children, before the age of three, as delays in their ability to socially interact and communicate. There are actually several types of autism, which are referred to as "autism spectrum disorders." All these disorders are characterized by varying degrees of impairment in communication skills and social interactions, and restricted, repetitive and stereotyped patterns of behavior. Autistic children usually appear to completely lack interest in other people, and seem to have enormous difficulty learning basic social skills. Signs of the disorder are often apparent in the first few months of life, as many autistic children seem indifferent to other people, not making eye contact or participating in social interactions that healthy children naturally engage in.

For reasons that no one understands, boys are four times more likely to have autism than girls. A child with autism may appear to develop normally and then withdraw and become indifferent to social interactions. Children with autism often avoid eye contact with other people and may even fail to respond to someone saying their name. They have great difficulty interpreting what other people are thinking or feeling because they generally don't understand social cues, such as the tone of one's voice or facial expressions. Autistic children don't watch other people's faces for clues about appropriate behavior and they seem to lack empathy.

Conventional medicine has little to offer people suffering from autism and the standard medical treatments are largely ineffective. The standard treatment for autism generally involves a combination of therapies, including occupational and physical therapy, behavior modification, communication therapy, dietary modifications, and a wide array of powerful but largely ineffective medications, including antidepressants, tranquilizers, stimulants, and antipsychotic medications. Most people with autism undergoing traditional therapies show little improvement and new treatments are desperately needed.

One promising new avenue of research that may one day provide treatment for adult autism involves the use of a psychoactive substance derived from nutmeg called MDMA (methylenedioxymethamphetamine), within the context of a psychotherapeutic setting, which has been reported to produce lasting feelings of empathy in some people. Numerous reports from people who have used MDMA report increased sociability and strong feelings of empathy that last long after the psychoactive effect of the substance wears off. There has been substantial interest in using MDMA as a possible treatment for less severe cases of adult autism because two of the hallmarks of the disorder are an inability to communicate socially and a lack of empathy.

David Jentsch at the UCLA Center for Autism is currently running a pilot project called "Towards a Neurochemistry of Sociability," to determine the effects of MDMA on the transmission of a key neurochemical in the brain called "vasopressin" as it relates to rat brain models of autism.[8] Vasopressin is known to mediate rodent sociability, and the study is designed to evaluate the effects of MDMA on social reinforcement in a mutant rat that is deficient in vasopressin secretion and that shows abnormal social recognition, like someone with autism. According to Dr. Jentsch, these pilot data are necessary to understand the neurochemistry of social reinforcement, and they may generate insights into the etiology and treatment of autistic spectrum disorders.

MAPS (The Multidisciplinary Association for Psychedelic Studies) also recently awarded a grant for a project that will use the internet to search for reports from people with a high-functioning form of autism called "Asperger's syndrome" who have found MDMA to be helpful in their learning to cope more effectively in social situations.[9] If they find enough reports this may become a new area of research. Finding novel treatments for autism is especially important because the number of reported cases appears to be on the rise.

In recent years there has been a large increase in the number of diagnosed cases of autism throughout the world.[10] The reasons for this are heavily debated by physicians, researchers, and parents with autistic children. The U.S. Centers for Disease Control estimates that the prevalence of autism disorders to be somewhere between one out of every five hundred births to one out of every hundred sixty-six births. Some epidemiologists argue that this increase in reported cases is primarily due to a broadening of the diagnostic criteria, reclassifications, or societal factors such as increased public awareness.

However, a substantial number of epidemiologists think the reason is environmental and research appears to confirm this.[11] A large-scale, comprehensive study—called the Autism Phenome Project—conducted by a team of physicians and scientific researchers at the University of California at Davis' MIND Institute is currently underway, and results from the pilot study appear to confirm that the increase in reported cases of autism has an environmental origin.[12] Results from the pilot study support the claim that the reported increase in autism is quite real, and substantial, even after accounting for changes in diagnostic criteria.

What Causes Autism?

One leading theory as to the neurological cause of autism attempts to trace its origin to a defect in what are called "mirror neurons," specialized neurons in the brain that are normally activated when we are observing other people.[13] In healthy people, mirror neurons are thought to play a significant role in social learning and in the general comprehension of other people's actions. While no one knows for sure exactly what causes mirror neurons to become defective—and it appears that the disorder may actually have multiple causes, including a large genetic component—we do have evidence that the worldwide increase in reported cases of autism is due to environmental influences.

Regardless of the precise neurological etiology, some people appear to have a greater genetic vulnerability to autism and a recent environmental change appears to be causing a sharp rise in the prevalence of the disorder among those who are most vulnerable. Desperate for clues, it seems, some researchers have blamed the increase in autism on excessive television viewing by children.[14] Television does cause neurochemical and brain wave frequency changes in the brain, and the long-term effects of watching television, or interacting with computers, is unknown. However, it seems unlikely that this is at the root of a disorder that is often witnessed in the first few months of birth.

A leading theory as to the cause of autism is directly related to the primary theme of this book, and the evidence appears to be supporting it more and more—that the primary reason why autism rates are increasing is because of the abundance of toxins and heavy metals in our food and environment. Some researchers have proposed the possible role of vaccines,[15] which—we learned in chapter 2—sometimes use mercury as a preservative, which can cause brain damage.

As I mentioned, there is also a large genetic component to autism. There is about a sixty percent concordance rate for autism among identical (monozygotic) twins, while non-identical twins and other siblings only exhibit about four percent concordance rates. Some people, it seems, are simply more vulnerable genetically to developing autism and my coauthor and I believe that these people are like canaries in the coal mines, alerting us to the fact that something is seriously wrong with our environment.

Another important theory regarding the cause of autism is related to what are known as "excitotoxins," chemicals that can damage brain tissue, which will be discussed in the next section. In my coauthor's previous book, *The Puzzle of Autism: Putting It All Together*, he reports that the protocol that he helped to develop for treating autism, based on lowering excitotoxin levels, has been remarkably effective.[16] A summary of the basic protocol and findings will be discussed here.

I was also able to speak with some of the parents who experienced success in treating their autistic children using this protocol and will provide some highlights from my interviews with them. For example one mother described the positive changes she witnessed in her child by saying, "Eye contact is fantastic. She just gazes at me all the time."

The Role of Excitotoxins in Our Diet

Understanding how Dr. Gordon's protocol for treating autism works requires that a few terms and metabolic processes first be explained. These are excitotoxins, methylation cycles, and genetic testing. Let's start by discussing the role that excitotoxins play in autism.

We learned at the beginning of this chapter that neurons communicate with one another using chemical messengers called "neurotransmitters." There are many dozens of known neurotransmitters—and there are likely many more waiting to be discovered—but they are all generally classified as being of two basic types: excitatory and inhibitory. (In some cases the same neurotransmitter can have both excitatory and inhibitory properties, depending on where and when in the brain it is released, but for discussion purposes we needn't worry about that now.) Excitatory neurotransmitters—such as dopamine—excite, speed up, or accelerate neural processes. Inhibitory neurotransmitters—such as serotonin—do exactly the opposite; they inhibit, calm, or slow down neural processes.

Glutamate is the primary excitatory neurotransmitter in the brain, and it is essential for learning and memory, although too much of it can be dangerous. Glutamate is also the metabolic precursor to GABA—one of the primary inhibitory neurotransmitters—that calms the nervous system and is essential for speech. The balance between the excitatory glutamate and the inhibitory GABA in the brain works something like a see saw; as the level of one neurotransmitter goes up the level of the other goes down, and vice versa.

When the brain is functioning normally, excess levels of glutamate will be converted to GABA, and the brain naturally cycles between periods of excitation and inhibition. However, according to Dr. Gordon, there seems to be a "disconnect" in this process for autistic children so that the excitatory neurotransmission is high and the calming neurotransmission is low. When conditions occur that throw off this delicate balance, then high levels of glutamate can accumulate in the brain while the levels of

GABA remain exceedingly low.

There is evidence, which will be discussed in the next chapter, that chronic viral infections may be related to this disconnect between glutamate and GABA. Interestingly, vitamin B-6 is used as a cofactor by the enzyme that is responsible for converting glutamate to GABA, and supplementation with this vitamin has been a long-standing part of some treatments for autism.

This problem of converting glutamate to GABA is dramatically compounded by the fact that most people have too much glutamate in their diet. Chemically, glutamate is an amino acid and it is commonly used as a food additive in the form of monosodium glutamate (MSG), because it excites our taste buds. We actually have specific taste buds for MSG, which is completely natural. MSG is found in a form of seaweed called kombu and has been used as a flavor enhancer in Japan for thousands of years.

But too much MSG can be dangerous because it can overexcite neurons to death. This is why it is so concerning that today in America, and around the world, MSG is added to most fast foods, frozen foods, ready-made dinners, soups, chips, and canned goods. It is often disguised in foods and sometimes appears in the ingredients as natural flavorings, spices, or hydrolyzed vegetable protein. Each of these ingredients may contain anywhere from twelve to forty percent MSG.

Two other amino acids—cysteine and aspartate (NutraSweet™)—are commonly used as food additives, and like glutamate, act as excitatory neurotransmitters that can cause brain damage when they become overly abundant in the nervous system. These excitatory neurotransmitters are sometimes referred to as "excitotoxins" because too many of them in the brain can cause neurons to die. Excitotoxins can excite neurons to death if their levels are not regulated properly.

For example, too much glutamate in the brain triggers an inflammatory process that results in the death of neurons due to a major influx of calcium into the cells. There are currently large amounts of these excitotoxins in our food supply and my coauthor believes that this is a big part of what is causing the increasing reports of autism around the world. Evidence to support this position comes from the reports that symptoms of autism decrease when excitotoxins levels are reduced in the brain. (An excellent source for learning more about excitotoxins is Russell Blaylock's book *Excitotoxins: The Taste that Kills*.)

When I spoke with Leslie Hamud, who is the mother of two autistic children, she told me that changing her children's diet—so as to eliminate the majority of excitotoxins—made a significant difference in her children's behavior. Leslie said, "When I changed their diet, all of a sudden, they became less 'spacey.' As the MSG and other excitotoxins in their food were diminished, that 'spaciness' improved. They developed a better ability to focus, to listen to your words, and take directions. And, gradually, as we continued to support the body and methylation pathways, all the way down the line things improved." (The full interview that I did with Leslie appears as Appendix B in the back of this book.)

Leslie brings up an important topic—methylation pathways. According to my coauthor, methylation pathways and methylation cycles are essential to understanding the puzzle of autism.

What are Methylation Cycles?

Methylation cycles are chemical reactions used by the body to accomplish such tasks as turning on genes or activating enzymes, and there are hundreds of different types of methylation reactions in the body. A "methyl" group consists of one carbon atom connected to three hydrogen atoms. Methylation is simply the process of adding or subtracting a methyl group to or from a chemical compound. When some compounds in the body receive a methyl group, this initiates a biochemical reaction—such as turning on a gene or activating an enzyme. When a methyl group is lost, then the reaction stops and the gene is turned off or the enzyme is deactivated.

Methylation reactions are important to this discussion for several reasons. They are responsible for turning on detoxification reactions in the body, so if there are disruptions in the methylation reactions then the toxic burden on the body can increase. Secondly, because the methylation cycles are essential for a number of critical reactions in the body, these are ideal pathways for intervention because certain supplements can be used to increase or decrease methylation reactions, thus turning on or turning off the expression of certain reactions in the body. It is also important to understand methylation cycles because mutations in the cycle may play an important role in the etiology of autism and other psychiatric disorders.

Mutations in the methylation pathways may limit the body's ability to synthesize the building blocks that organs need for repair and growth. They can weaken the body's ability to make the chemical precursors necessary for new DNA and RNA synthesis, which means that the body's ability to develop new cells is impaired. Because cells are continuously dying, the body needs to create millions of new cells every minute, and it relies upon DNA and RNA synthesis to accomplish this. According to Dr. Gordon, these types of methylation pathway mutations would result in a decreased level of new T cell synthesis, which is an essential part of the immune system and is necessary for the body to respond to viral infection. T cells are needed to create antibody-producing cells in the body, and antibodies are our primary line of defense against infectious pathogens.

As we learned in the last chapter, there is a growing body of evidence, and a compelling theoretical foundation, to support the notion that many common chronic diseases—which are thought to be caused primarily by a combination of defective genes and/or an unhealthy lifestyle— might actually be caused by an infectious pathogen, such as a virus or a form of bacteria, that doesn't have an acute phase of harm.[17] Some evolutionary biologists are making a strong case for the idea that many of the supposedly benign pathogens and microbes that chronically infect our bodies may not be quite as benign as has been previously thought, and Dr. Gordon thinks that they may play a role in autism.

Because mutations in the methylation pathways can limit cell growth in the body, this may result in a reduced number of pathogen-fighting T cells. If the body produces too few T cells then the immune system suffers and pathogens can thrive. The damage that seemingly benign bacteria, viruses, and fungi do when they chronically infect the body is largely unknown, although evidence is beginning to accumulate that some of these chronic infections may cause significant damage to our health over time. If pathogens play a role in autism due to lower T cells in the immune system, then an effective treatment could be developed by addressing the mutations in the methylation pathways—and this is exactly what my coauthor has been working on, with very effective results.

So, according to Dr. Gordon, one of the most important first steps in treating autism involves identifying mutations in the methylation pathways, and this can be done through genomic testing.

The Importance of Genomic Testing

Many risk factors can be derived from doing a genetic analysis. With the completion of the Human Genome Project, and the accompanying evolution of molecular biology techniques, genomic tests are now available that can examine the minute differences between each person's DNA. Genomic testing thus enables individuals to evaluate and address the genetic component of a disease that is caused by multiple factors.

Currently, genomic tests are available that can identify a number of underlying genetic susceptibilities based on variations that are found in the genome. Because there is a large genetic component to autism, genetic testing appears to be essential for treating it. The most important way to evaluate the genetic contribution of a multifactorial disease like autism is to take advantage of the new methodologies that allow for personalized genetic screening.

Problems in the methylation pathways can be revealed through genetic testing, and this is why doing a DNA analysis is especially important for treating autism. Dr. Gordon has learned that a range of possible mutations, in a variety of genes in the methylation pathway, can compromise its function and serve as a predisposing factor for autism. By analyzing genetic data from over five hundred children, Dr. Gordon has learned that virtually a hundred percent of these individuals have one or more mutations in particular genes that are involved in this pathway.

Having a genetic vulnerability in the methylation cycle pathways serves as a risk factor for autism, as well as a number of serious health conditions, including other neurological disorders, cardiovascular disease, and cancer. Some researchers even think that mutations in the methylation cycle pathways may accelerate the aging process itself.

Dr. Gordon thinks that the methylation pathways are the ideal pathways to focus on for "nutrigenomic analysis" and supplementation. Nutrigenomics is the prescription of foods and nutrient supplements based on analysis of individual genetic risk factors. Many physicians and researchers believe that nutrigenomic analysis will be a standard part of every medical checkup in the future, providing each patient with a detailed list of tailored suggestions and nutritional recommendations.

So now that we understand the role that excitotoxins play in autism, how mutations in the methylation cycles make certain individuals more vulnerable to the effects of certain pathogens and heavy metals, and the importance of genomic testing in identifying genetic vulnerabilities, we can now begin to piece together a protocol for treating this illness that devastates the lives of so many people.

Putting the Puzzle of Autism Together

There are three primary steps to Dr. Gordon's protocol for treating autism.

The first step involves removing excitotoxins from the diet because they are known to cause inflammation in the brain and neuron death. This requires that the foods mentioned above that contain MSG and other excitotoxins—such as many fast foods, frozen foods, ready-made dinners, soups, chips, and canned goods—be completely eliminated from the diet. Then Dr. Gordon uses nutritional support to lay the groundwork for repairing damaged brain cells and generating new neural growth. This is accomplished with a variety of herbs, vitamins, and nutritional supplements.

The second step involves using EDTA chelation therapy and other detoxification methods to remove toxins and pathogens from the body, which will be discussed more below. The third step in the program is designed to support nerve growth and a process known as "myelination." Myelination is the formation of a fatty, electrically-insulating layer around nerve fibers called a "myelin sheath." A myelin sheath is like the rubber layer insulating household electrical wiring, and it insulates the electrical transmission of neurons in the brain and nervous system.

Demyelination is the loss of the myelin sheath that insulates the nerves. This is the hallmark of certain neurodegenerative autoimmune diseases—such as multiple sclerosis—and the immune system often plays a role in the demyelination that is associated with such diseases. However, heavy metal poisoning may also lead to demyelination, and even very small amounts of mercury have been shown to be particularly destructive to nerve sheaths. When myelin degrades, conduction of electrical signals along the nerve can be impaired or lost, and the nerve eventually withers.

According to Dr. Gordon, it can take up to nine months to remyelinate the nerves that have been demyelinated from viruses, metals, and other heavily destructive assaults on our body's systems—but the nervous system will regenerate and grow healthy myelinated brain cells with time. Because the methylation pathway is also connected to the pathways that manufacture neurotransmitters, brain chemistry begins to return to normal as autistic patients detoxify their bodies and fortify themselves with nutritional supplements.

For more information on my coauthor's protocol for treating autism see his book *The Puzzle of Autism: Putting It All Together*, the accompanying *Beyond Autism Conference* DVD set, and his Web site: www.gordonresearch.com. Although the details of this treatment program are too lengthy to be included here, it is important for our discussion to emphasize that an essential part of this treatment involves EDTA chelation therapy and other detoxification strategies.

Autism & EDTA Chelation Therapy

It's interesting to point out that some of the symptoms seen in autism resemble aspects of heavy metal toxicity, which suggests a connection between the two. For example, in chapter 2 we learned that the symptoms of lead poisoning include serious learning disabilities, reduced intelligence, and neurological problems.

My coauthor reports that heavy metal chelation and detoxification methods have proven successful in helping to treat and reverse the symptoms of autism. These reports are supported by the accumulating evidence that levels of lead and other heavy metals tend to increase in the urine of autistic children as their symptoms tend to decrease when they are treated with EDTA chelation therapy. Dr. Gordon believes that this is because heavy metals interfere with the methylation cycles and that EDTA chelation therapy is essential for treating autism.

Another piece to this complex puzzle emerges with the understanding that copper sometimes replaces zinc in the body and this suppresses GABA production in the brain. These disruptions in zinc/copper ratios have been well characterized by Dr. William Walsh, Director of Research at the Pfeiffer Treatment Center in Illinois, and this ties into the glutamate and GABA imbalances associated with autism. The successful use of EDTA chelation therapy with autistic children may be partially due to the fact that it helps to decrease copper levels in the brain. This releases the GABA from copper suppression, and helps to balance the zinc/copper ratio in the body.

For numerous reasons, EDTA chelation therapy appears to be an essential tool for treating autism, cerebrovascular disease, and neurodegenerative disorders such as senile dementia and Alzheimer's disease because it removes toxins and improves circulation in the brain. It may also be effective in treating some forms of depression (especially postpartum depression) as many people report a strong antidepressant effect from EDTA chelation therapy.

In another study at the Pfeiffer Treatment Center, Dr. Walsh found that elevated levels of copper in a new mother's body may contribute to postpartum depression. Dr. Walsh studied the medical records of fourteen thousand women and found that women with a history of postpartum depression had significantly higher blood copper levels compared to those without depression. Postpartum depression affects about four hundred thousand women in the United States, with debilitating symptoms, including depressed moods, low energy and little appetite, sleep disturbances, and a reduced interest in normally enjoyable activities. EDTA chelation therapy may be effective in treating postpartum depression that results from elevated copper levels because it helps to decrease copper levels in the brain.

EDTA chelation therapy serves as a multipurpose tool for repairing a malfunctioning brain and treating mental illness. Although it has been shown to be efficacious in treating numerous psychiatric disorders (especially those associated with heavy metal toxicity), it also appears to effectively improve cognitive performance in healthy individuals. Let's take a look at how we can use EDTA—and a few other valuable substances—to enhance mental health and improve the performance of a healthy human brain.

Smart Drugs, Herbs, & Nutrients

EDTA is sometimes referred to as a "nootropic" or "smart drug" because it increases blood flow to the brain, and there are many reports that it can improve attention, concentration, memory, and cognitive performance in general. "Nootropics" are a class of drugs that have been shown to improve cognition and mental clarity. The more media-friendly term "smart drug" was coined by my colleague, John Morgenthaler, to refer to this new class of pharmaceuticals that is unusually safe and may be able to increase intelligence by improving certain brain functions. Some of the substances, like EDTA, also increase blood flow to the brain. For example, the ergot-derived "smart drug" Hydergine and the herb ginkgo biloba have also been shown to improve cerebral blood flow, memory, and mental concentration. Both are widely used around the world for treating neurodegenerative disorders.[18]

Hydergine was specifically developed because of its ability to improve peripheral circulation and cerebral function in the control of geriatric disorders, and it has proven to be an effective treatment for these indications.[19] Hydergine was the first drug to show efficacy as a treatment for Alzheimer's disease and dementias. Today Hydergine is widely used as a treatment for senility, age-related cognitive decline, and a number of other problems. Extensive research has revealed a plethora of brain-boosting and anti-aging benefits that it has to offer. Hydergine is one of the most tested pharmaceuticals ever developed and it has proven to be beneficial and nontoxic in numerous studies.[20]

Studies indicate that Hydergine has the ability to enhance memory and learning.[21] It improves a range of cognitive abilities, such as concentration and recall and helps to prevent damage to brain cells from insufficient oxygen. A number of studies even suggest that Hydergine may be able to help reverse existing damage to brain cells.[22] Some of Hydergine's cognitive enhancement may be due to the fact that it increases oxygen and blood flow to the brain because it's a mild vasodilator. It also enhances brain cell metabolism and mitochondrial metabolism. Hydergine's ability to improve cell metabolism inspired a team of Italian researchers to study how it effects the intracellular features of rat mitochondria, structures within cells that produce energy in the form of ATP by respiratory metabolism. In these studies Hydergine not only increased the volume of the mitochondria, it also reduced their size, which is similar to the more efficient mitochondria in younger animals.[23]

Another important cognitive enhancer that improves circulation to the brain (and throughout the body) comes from the ginkgo biloba tree. Ginkgo biloba has been cultivated in China for over a thousand years and some of the trees planted at Buddhist temples in Asia are thought to be over fifteen hundred years old. Extracts of the ginkgo biloba leaves contain what are known as "flavonoid glycosides" and "terpenoids," and studies show that these substances can improve circulation and have cognitive-enhancing properties.[24] This is why ginkgo biloba has been widely used as a memory enhancer in healthy individuals, as well as a treatment for age-related cognitive decline, memory disorders, and vertigo.

Ginkgo biloba appears to have three basic effects on the human body. It improves blood flow to most tissues and organs, including microcirculation in small capillaries. It acts as an antioxidant and protects against oxidative cell damage from free radicals. It also blocks many of the effects of platelet aggregation and blood clotting that have been related to the development of a number of cardiovascular, renal, respiratory and neurological disorders. Ginkgo biloba has also been used as an effective treatment for intermittent claudication (leg cramping). Studies indicate that ginkgo biloba shows some promise in the treatment of Alzheimer's disease, although further research in this area is badly needed. Ginkgo biloba, like EDTA, is non-patentable, and because of this pharmaceutical companies aren't terribly motivated to fund the needed research into its effects.

Like these smart drugs and herbs, EDTA may also be useful for improving memory and enhancing concentration in healthy individuals. Although scientific studies demonstrating more of EDTA's brain-boosting effects are badly needed, we know that it increases circulation to the brain, and there is no shortage of anecdotal reports regarding its ability to improve mental performance. I can personally attest to this and I simply would not be writing this book if I hadn't experienced these effects firsthand myself. It may be important to point out that many personal anecdotes that I've read report that nootropic substances tend to be more effective when they are taken together, and that there is a synergistic effect that comes from combining various cognitive enhancers. For more information on combining cognitive enhancers, and about smart drugs in general, please see John Morgenthaler and Ward Dean's excellent books *Smart Drugs and Nutrients* and *Smart Drugs II*.[25]

The desire to increase human intelligence is part of a long evolutionary trend on this planet, and this is why we tend to perceive intelligence as being a sexually attractive trait. All human cultures generally value education and strive to accumulate knowledge—first through books and then through electronic mediums—because throughout evolution brain size has generally been increasing and higher intelligence has generally been favored by natural selection. The accelerating expansion of higher intelligence is one obvious trend in evolution; another is an increase in life span. A lengthening of the early developmental stages in an animal's growth, and an increase in the number of years lived, are strongly established patterns in biological evolution.

As our species learns how to survive for longer and longer periods of time, it appears that our desire for even longer life naturally increases, and humanity's quest for immortality is at least as ancient as history itself. The oldest surviving story ever written—*The Epic of Gilgamesh*—is about a king's search for eternal life. This ancient quest for everlasting life has evolved over time into the scientific study of longevity and, more recently, into life extension research. As we will learn in the next chapter—which is on pathogens, disease prevention, and anti-aging— EDTA chelation therapy not only appears to extend life due to its ability to prevent disease, but also because it may help to slow down and reverse aspects of the aging process itself.

Chapter 5

DISEASE PREVENTION AND ANTI-AGING

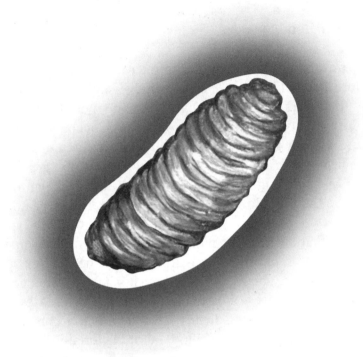

According to most healthcare experts—and conventional wisdom—genes, diet, lifestyle, and environmental pollutants are the primary factors in determining whether or not people develop cardiovascular disease, most forms of cancer, Alzheimer's disease, and other common chronic diseases. However, a number of prominent evolutionary biologists think otherwise. Leading the pack is Paul Ewald, who has proposed a compelling theory for explaining the basis for many deadly diseases that plague the human species.

In his eye-opening book *Plague Time*, Ewald presents an abundance of largely ignored evidence that makes a strong case for the notion that seemingly benign, slowly acting, chronically infecting pathogens—without acute phases of harm—may be at the root cause of many deadly ailments that we erroneously think are due to genetic or environmental factors.[1] In other words, Ewald believes that the most common chronic diseases that kill us—heart disease, breast cancer, prostate cancer, Alzheimer's disease, etc.—are likely caused by a virus or some form of bacteria that's already living inside of us.

We Are Their Food Source

Our bodies are simply swarming with microbes, bacteria, viruses, and fungi. More than half of every person's body weight is made up of these microscopic critters. Each person carries around more foreign cells than cells of their own body. Some forms of bacteria, such as those found in our gut, are not only helpful, but necessary for digestion. However, most of these microscopic critters in our bodies are invaders, parasites not symbiotes, and the long-term consequences of having them live inside of us   where they are slowly eating away at us—is largely unknown.

Ewald thinks that our focus in medicine on acute infections that require immediate attention has blinded us from seeing the long-term dangers of chronic, seemingly benign infections. This has already been proven true in a number of cases. We now know that some diseases that were long thought to have genetic, dietary, lifestyle, or environmental causes are actually usually due primarily to viral or bacterial infections. Some examples are cervical cancer, which is usually caused by the human papilloma virus, and stomach ulcers, which are largely caused by the *h. pylori* bacterium.

The compelling nature of Ewald's theory is strengthened by its evolutionary perspective. It makes evolutionary sense that microbes who use us as their food supply would evolve to do so in such a manner that allows them to proliferate as much as possible, as stealthily as possible—to their advantage at our expense. Animal immune systems and quickly evolving pathogens are involved in an ancient competition that stretches far back into our evolutionary past. They have been competing for millions of years, and this long-standing competition is likely to continue for quite some time into the future, so it seems wise to learn how to best adapt ourselves to living with these tenacious microscopic critters.

It is important to realize that the application of evolutionary principles does not lead to the conclusion that all pathogens evolve toward benignness, as was previously thought. Pathogens simply evolve in such a way as to maximize their consumption of people as much as possible, without killing off each individual before they can infect a new host. For this reason, Ewald advocates a new discipline called "evolutionary epistemology," which applies evolutionary principles to the study and treatment of infectious disease.

The consequences of the indiscriminate and widespread use of antibiotics as a preventative for infectious disease serves as an example of how not paying attention to evolutionary principles can lead to greater problems in the long-run. In this particular case powerful and deadly strains of antibiotic-resistance bacteria have been created through our ignorant and widespread use of antibiotics. These deadly strains of super-bacteria are now starting to seriously threaten our health.

Although better hygiene has largely eliminated the means of transport-ation for most of the deadly microbes that cause acute damage in First World countries, plenty of microbes still regard First World inhabitants as their primary source of food. The chronic infections from these organisms have been largely overlooked by medicine, and this, Ewald believes, may hold the key to understanding many of the chronic diseases that plague modern humans.

If Ewald's theory is correct—and many experts agree that, at the very least, it certainly deserves serious attention—then we need to take action. In a very literal sense we are the food supply for these other organisms. We are all like the victims in the science fiction film *Invasion of the Body Snatchers*, where alien invaders grow genetic replicas of people in plant-like pods in order to replace them. Microscopic alien invaders have been feeding off the human species since the beginning of time and this provides yet another compelling reason why EDTA chelation therapy is one of the most important things that we can be doing to help improve our health.

Some of these pathogens are known to result in chronic infections that can cause heavy metals to accumulate in the body. EDTA not only helps to remove these heavy metals that accumulate, but it has also been shown to have powerful antioxidant and antiviral properties, which we will discuss—but, first, let's take a look at how our immune system operates.

The Immune System

Our bodies are constantly under attack by microorganisms—such as bacteria, viruses, and fungi. The immune system is like the police force that protects our bodies from these undersized terrorist invaders. The immune system is a network of mechanisms in the body that work to prevent infection by identifying and killing pathogens—ranging from viruses and bacteria to parasitic worms. Most people don't know that the immune system is actually an information-processing system—similar to the brain—which recognizes and remembers pathogens, learns from its experience, and actually makes decisions that effect whether or not we live or die.

The immune system's ability to detect pathogens is complicated, and distinguishing these foreign invaders from the body's normal cells and tissues isn't always easy. This is because pathogens are continuously adapting to our defenses against them, and they're always evolving new ways to outsmart our immune systems so that they can infect our bodies.

The immune system consists of many types of proteins, cells, organs, and tissues, which interact in an elaborate network, and adapt over time to recognize particular pathogens more efficiently. The adaptation process creates immunological memories and allows for more effective protection during future encounters with these pathogens. This process of acquired immunity is the basis of vaccination.

Environmental pollutants and heavy metals are known to impair virtually all aspects of immune function.[2] Because the atomic structure of lead and zinc are so closely related to each other, as we raise the levels of lead we start plugging lead into key enzyme functions in our immune system that normally zinc would have fulfilled. This creates a vicious cycle. Our immune systems become impaired due to heavy metal contamination, which makes them less efficient at fighting off pathogens. As pathogen levels rise so do levels of heavy metals, because some types of bacteria cause heavy metals to accumulate. More heavy metals in our body then causes the immune system to suffer so pathogen levels continue to rise, and the cycle continues.

Pathogens interact with heavy metals in the body in a variety of dangerous ways. For example, the mercury in dental fillings is converted to methyl mercury by bacteria. Methyl mercury is a potent neurotoxin that is easily absorbed by nerve cells. Mercury in the nervous system interferes with energy production in individual cells, and the cell's ability to detoxify itself becomes impaired. Our immune systems are under continuous assault from environmental pollutants and they can use all the help that they can get. EDTA chelation therapy is incredibly effective in this regard, because not only does it help to remove heavy metals and restore immune function, it also has antiviral and antioxidant properties of its own.

EDTA's Antiviral & Antioxidant Properties

EDTA has been shown to have both antiviral and antioxidant properties. A virus is simply a strand of genetic material wrapped in a protein coat. It's debatable whether or not that tiny strand of DNA or RNA should even be considered a life form, yet those little buggers have the power to completely hijack the cells in your body and turn them into factories that produce nothing but more viruses. Our immune systems learn to recognize viruses and develop antibodies against them.

Vaccinations help the immune system to recognize pathogens; they're like mug shots given to the police detectives of our immune systems so they know who to watch out for. But viruses are continuously evolving and changing their tactics. Antibiotics, which are very effective in treating bacterial infections, have no effect whatsoever on viral infections. There are some antiviral prescription medications, such as acyclovir, famciclovir and valacyclovir, but these pharmaceutical drugs are not terribly effective on many viruses and they can have serious side-effects. Common outbreaks of viruses such as herpes, influenza, HIV, and the common cold demonstrate that we need a whole lot more help to deal with them.

A number of studies have shown that EDTA has antiviral properties.

An early study done in 1955 by Vincent Groupe and others at Rutgers University demonstrated that chelated cobalt protects against the influenza virus.[3] Dr. Groupe and his colleagues showed that cobalt chelated with EDTA will inhibit the multiplication of the influenza virus. Then a German study in 1982 by Wunderlich and Sydow demonstrated that the exposure of various mammalian retroviruses to the chelating agents EDTA or EGTA—in millimolar concentrations—resulted in a partial disintegration of viral membranes.[4] Other studies have shown that EDTA has a mild antiviral effect on its own, but it dramatically increases the effectiveness of other antiviral treatments.

"EDTA's antiviral activity is important," Dr. Gordon says, "because we're now learning that heart disease doesn't have much to do with cholesterol—like everybody has been told because it sells lots of lipitor and other drugs—but, rather, has much more to do with inflammation. Inflammation is due to many things, but one of the things that it is clearly due to is our low level infections due to the total burden of pathogens. This includes chlamydia, Epstein-Barr, herpes, mycoplasma incognito, SV40, and the list goes on and on. No one today is free of these infections. Paul Ewald documents the fact that doctors do not even diagnose the chlamydia in everybody today because it is so ubiquitous and you can't cure it."

In addition to all those viruses, the body is also swarming with chronic bacterial infections. Bacteria are tiny one-celled organisms and antibiotics will usually kill them—unless they've adapted to the antibiotic through misuse. But even if the bacteria didn't develop a resistance to antibiotics, taking an antibiotic regularly to simply lower these chronic infections in the body wouldn't be terribly helpful because the drugs would have serious side effects, like killing important bacteria that the body is symbiotic with and putting the body's chemistry out of balance. Then, of course, the moment that one stops taking an antibiotic the bacterial infections would simply return.

EDTA works as a mild antiviral treatment but its antioxidant properties have been shown to be quite powerful,[5] and this also helps the body to fight off infections. Antioxidants are essential for the body to be able to slow down the damage caused by what are known as "free radicals." Free radicals are not anything like free-spirited Yippies. Rather, they are highly reactive atoms or molecules with unpaired electrons. Free radicals can cause substantial oxidative damage to the body and are thought to be one of the primary causes of aging. Because free radicals are necessary for normal metabolism, the body uses antioxidants to minimize free radical-induced damage. Antioxidants provide free radicals with a paired electron that thereby neutralizes it and prevents it from causing any further damage.

All metals catalyze free radicals in the body. The antioxidant effect of EDTA is directly due to the fact that free metals cause free radicals and EDTA's antioxidant effect has been well documented. "So if you really want a powerful antioxidant, then EDTA would truly be strongest of them all because it has the ability to tie up every metal," Dr. Gordon said. EDTA will tie up the metals so that they're no longer free. At the atomic level, an atom of lead, copper, or iron is surrounded by what's called a "hexidentate" molecule, and this dovetails perfectly with the molecular configuration of EDTA. It's the way that all of the molecules of EDTA line up.

EDTA functions as an antioxidant, preventing free radicals from injuring blood vessel walls and other tissues in the body,[6] but EDTA chelation therapy isn't the only tool that we have to strengthen the immune system.

Other Tools That Enhance the Immune System

In chapter 2 we discussed garlic's powerful detoxifying properties and that it contains allicin, which is a strong antibiotic. We also discussed vitamin C's antioxidant properties and how these properties can help to prevent many chronic diseases. Garlic and vitamin C are also important to our discussion here because these supplements can be used to help aid the immune system in lowering the body's total burden of pathogens. Some of the other important supplements that are pertinent to our discussion on disease prevention are colloidal silver, carnivora, and oil of oregano.

Colloidal Silver

Colloidal silver is a heterogeneous mixture of extremely tiny, evenly distributed silver particles in water. It is well established that colloidal silver has powerful antimicrobial properties. For over a hundred years prior to the discovery of antibiotics colloidal silver was used on external wounds and burns to treat infection. It can be used to keep water pure and drinkable over a long period of time as high concentrations of colloidal silver kill bacteria and other microbes. An abundance of new evidence demonstrates that colloidal silver has strong antibiotic and antiviral properties, and that it can be used as an effective tool for lowering the body's burden of pathogens.

There is, however, some concern that, in rare cases, the ingestion of colloidal silver in large quantities, or over long periods of time, may carry a risk of argyria, a non-reversible condition in which the skin becomes discolored and turns blue-gray. The continued ingestion of more than a gram of accumulated silver, or five milligrams per day, may result in this rare condition, which is not serious and has no physiological implications. However, if one is careful to use only properly produced (five parts per million) colloidal silver then argyria is virtually impossible. According to Dr. Gordon, one tablespoon of colloidal silver with the proper safety ratios can be taken daily for thirty years without any risk of argyria, and even a pint can be taken daily for up to six months without the risk of turning blue.

Carnivora

Another substance important to our discussion is Carnivora. Carnivora is an extract of the venus flytrap plant—a fascinating carnivorous plant that catches small insects in its quickly snapping traps and then slowly digests them with powerful enzymes. Carnivora contains seventeen important compounds with antimicrobial and immune system enhancing properties. These valuable compounds in the venus flytrap are a result of its advanced immune system, which is unusually effective at distinguishing between harmful intruders and its own cells. The plant only digests the undeveloped and undifferentiated cells of its prey and these type of cells are very similar to the pathogens that invade the human body—and proliferate as a result of exposure to environmental toxins, poor diets, and other dangerous health habits.

Carnivora supplementation can not only help to support the immune system by fortifying the body's own defense mechanisms, and blocking viral entry into our cells, it also acts directly on the pathogens themselves and kills them. Carnivora has been shown to contain strong detoxification and antimicrobial properties.[7] It helps to prevent infections, as well as DNA damage, and benefits the modulation of the immune system. However, whether or not vegetarians can ingest these carnivorous plant extracts and remain true "vegetarians" remains more of a philosophical question than a biological one.

Oil of Oregano

Oil of oregano is an extract from the oregano plant, a member of the mint family, with extraordinary properties. This is not to be confused with the common oregano found in your kitchen spice cupboard, which is usually marjoram (*Origanum majorana*) rather than true oregano (*Origanum vulgare*). True oregano has potent antioxidant properties and the oil of oregano has strong antiviral, antibacterial, and antifungal properties with no known side-effects. Oil pressed from oregano leaves contains an active compound called "carvacrol," which is a powerful antibiotic and may be an effective treatment against certain types of bacterial infections that are resistant to pharmaceutical antibiotics.

Georgetown University researchers have found that the oil of oregano appears to reduce bacterial infections "as effectively as traditional antibiotics,"[8] and the body of evidence for oregano oil as a major antibiotic is growing.[9,10,11] Oil of oregano, at relatively low doses, was found to be effective in treating *Staphylococcus* bacteria and was comparable in its germ-killing properties to antibiotic drugs such as streptomycin and penicillin.[12] Researchers at the University of Tennessee reported that, among the various plant oils that they tested, oil of oregano exhibited the greatest antibacterial action against common pathogenic germs such as Staph and E. coli.[13] British researchers have reported that oil of oregano has antibacterial activity against twenty-five different forms of bacteria,[14] and a clinical study in Italy has shown that it can be used to effectively treat intestinal parasites.[15]

As we discussed earlier in this chapter, the growing problem of bacteria that have evolved antibiotic resistance has health authorities concerned. Already various germs (particularly intestinal bacteria among hospitalized patients) are showing resistance to vancomycin, which is considered to be the most potent antibiotic available and is only used as a last resort. Because of this serious threat, which is escalating every day, it is important to point out that drug resistance does not develop against naturally occurring antibiotics such as the allicin in garlic or the carvacrol in oregano oil.

It is still not fully understood how allicin and carvacrol achieve their antibiotic action, but to date antibiotic resistance hasn't been observed with allicin, garlic's primary active ingredient, or with the carvacrol in oregano oil. These natural antibiotic processes aren't well understood because they haven't been carefully studied. Carvacrol appears to disrupt an important layer (lipopolysaccharide) in the cellular membrane of bacteria, and apparently, in general, the bacteria have great difficulty adapting to this because the conditions are so disruptive. This lack of antibiotic resistance has also been reported for colloidal silver, a substance in olive leaf extract called "oleuropein," and alcohol.

According to Ewald people should use alcohol-based cleaners to sterilize their hands and utensils rather than antibacterial soaps, which, over time, help to create more powerful strains of bacteria. I suspect that frogs and other amphibians—with their unusually permeable membranes, that allow water to easily flow through their skin—may hold many as yet undiscovered secrets applicable to novel antibiotic approaches. However, despite the widely publicized problem of a growing resistance to pharmaceutical antibiotics, the National Institutes of Health has yet to sponsor a human clinical study using any natural antibiotics.

Oil of oregano can be taken internally and applied topically, where its antimicrobial vapors will deeply penetrate skin tissue. Recent reports show that carvacrol from oregano oil is so powerful it even kills deadly anthrax spores, but it is also safe enough to be used as a treatment for common fungal infections like athlete's foot. It is reported to be effective against nail fungus and can often be as efficient as the pharmaceutical drug Lamisil®, without the dangerous side-effects that result from its toxic effect on the liver.

These supplements are effective tools for preventing and fighting disease. They can be used to help lower the body's total burden of pathogens, which helps to prevent many chronic diseases, but perhaps the ultimate form of disease prevention comes from slowing down the aging process itself. Let's take a look at how our bodies age and what we can do to help reverse it.

Slowing Down & Reversing the Aging Process

Is aging a disease? Some researchers think of aging as a disease that we all suffer from, while others see it as a natural and inevitable part of human development. However, regardless of whether or not aging itself is a (possibly curable) disease, it certainly increases the likelihood that one will develop problems with their body as time goes by, so it would be to everyone's advantage to learn how to slow down or reverse the aging process. But first, we need to know why we age and no one fully understands the process. Although there are some good theories of aging, and a lot of progress has been made in recent years, the aging process is still largely mysterious.

There are two prominent theories of aging that are important to our discussion. They are the cross-linking and free radical theories of aging. The cross-linking theory focuses on a process in the body called glycation, which is a chemical reaction between proteins and sugars that results in toxic products. These toxic products are thought to be one of the primary causes of aging. Glycation causes a process called "cross-linking," which is when two or more molecules become chemically joined with a covalent bond; i.e., when electrons are shared between them.

This sometimes results in the formation of abnormal chemical bonds between adjacent protein strands, which deforms them and impairs their function in the body. This is how much of what we observe as aging occurs. For example, age spots on the skin and cataracts in the eye, are caused by crosslinked proteins, as is a general loss of skin elasticity. The accumulation of crosslinked proteins can lead to cardiovascular disease, and all kinds of serious complications with the body. This is why too much sugar in one's diet can accelerate the aging process.

Two substances that are known to help prevent glycation in the body are an amino acid called L-carnosine and a pharmaceutical drug called aminoguanidine.

The other prominent theory of aging is the free radical theory. As we learned earlier, free radicals are highly reactive atoms or molecules with unpaired electrons that can cause substantial oxidative damage to the body. This damage is thought to be one of the primary causes of aging. Because free radicals are necessary for normal metabolism, the body uses antioxidants to minimize free radical-induced damage by preventing the oxidative degradation of other chemicals and helping to neutralize free radicals in the body. Environmental pollutants are known to dramatically increase the amount of free radicals in the body, so we need all the antioxidants that we can get. Some important antioxidants include vitamins C and E, carotenoids, alpha lipoic acid, coenzyme Q-10, ginkgo biloba, and melatonin. EDTA has also been shown to have strong antioxidant properties.

EDTA has other anti-aging properties besides helping to remove free radicals from the body;[17] it may also stimulate the activity of mitochondria in our cells, which produce energy in the form of ATP. One of the primary symptoms of aging is that one experiences less physical energy. Mitochondrial activity is known to decrease with age, and this is one of the primary reasons that people report having less and less energy as they get older. Mitochondria are structures within cells that produce energy by respiratory metabolism. EDTA is thought to stimulate mitochondrial activity, because lead is known to inhibit mitochondrial activity,[16] and this is probably one of the primary reasons why people who practice EDTA chelation therapy report having so much more energy as they get older.

Note: For readers who are interested in finding out more about aging research, one of the very best books on the subject is Aubrey de Grey's *Ending Aging* (St. Martin's Press, 2007). My previous book, *Mavericks of Medicine* (Smart Publications, 2006), contains an in-depth interview that I did with Dr. de Grey on the causes of aging, and what might be done to slow it down and reverse it.

Other Important Anti-Aging Agents

Some other important antiaging supplements include resveratrol, pueraria mirifica, deprenyl, melatonin, DHEA, and growth hormone (GH).

Longevity researchers have long known that caloric restriction can help to extend the maximum life span of laboratory animals. It's important to this discussion to understand the difference between maximum life span and average life span. Many factors can affect the average life span (or the "normal life expectancy") that an animal lives—genetics, diet, exercise, nutritional supplements, mental attitude, etc. However, even under the very best of conditions, there is an upper limit at which the longest-lived animals of a particular species can survive, and that is the animal's maximum life span. Extending maximum life span means extending the maximum number of years that the longest-lived members of a particular species have been known to attain.

The average life span of a human being is approximately seventy to eighty years, while the maximum life span is around a hundred twenty years. The caloric restriction studies are so impressive because they demonstrate a significant increase in the maximum life span of laboratory animals. These experiments have been successful with mammals from rats to monkeys, so there is good reason to suspect that caloric restriction would probably increase the maximum life span of human beings as well. Caloric restriction is defined as significantly reducing the amount of calories that an animal would eat, if given the option to eat as much as it likes, while making sure that all of its nutritional requirements are met.

However, as impressive as these studies are, many people view these findings with disappointment, because the idea of living longer, while being able to enjoy food less, doesn't sound very appealing. So it's been thrilling to discover that certain supplements and drugs—such as resveratrol and deprenyl—actually appear to mimic the effects of caloric restriction and also increase maximum life span.

Resveratrol

Resveratrol is botanical compound known as a polyphenol that has been shown to extend the life span of a number of different animal species.[18] It is found in a variety of different plants—including peanuts, pine nuts, raspberries, and cranberries—but is most well-known for being abundant in the skin of red grapes and as a constituent of red wine. Resveratrol is produced in the grape skin in response to a bacterial infection that affects the plant and it acts as a natural antibiotic. Polyphenols make up a large group of plant compounds and are broken down further into other chemical compounds—such as flavonoids and proanthocyanidins—which are known to be potent antioxidants.

It was initially thought that understanding the properties of resveratrol might help to explain the so-called "French paradox"—that the incidence of coronary heart disease is relatively low in southern France despite a high dietary intake of saturated fats. While a number of studies reported that the quantities of resveratrol found in red wine are not high enough to explain the "paradox," researchers did find that resveratrol has extraordinary health-enhancing properties. Some researchers believe that resveratrol works by mimicking the effects that one would get from practicing a calorically restricted diet, and that it activates the same genes that are triggered by caloric restriction.

A number of beneficial health effects have been reported from giving resveratrol to laboratory animals—such as anticancer, antiviral, neuroprotective, anti-aging, anti-inflammatory and life-prolonging effects. Johan Auwerx and colleagues at the Institute of Genetics and Molecular and Cell Biology in Illkirch, France, have found that resveratrol increases the activity of a protein called SIRT1,[19] and that resveratrol significantly increases the maximum life span of mice similar to caloric restriction. A recent study published in the science journal *Nature* by David Sinclair at Harvard University and others, showed that resveratrol significantly improves the health and survival of mice on a high-calorie diet.[20]

Sinclair and his colleagues showed that resveratrol actually shifts the physiology of middle-aged mice on a high-calorie diet towards that of mice on a standard diet and significantly increases their survival.

Resveratrol produces changes associated with longer life span—including increased insulin sensitivity, increased mitochondrial number, and improved motor function. Sinclair's study revealed that resveratrol opposed the effects of a high-calorie diet in a hundred forty-four out of a hundred fifty-three significantly altered biochemical pathways.

It's important to note that one study has shown that resveratrol also appears to have some mild MAO inhibition effects and that it may act as a noradrenaline and serotonin reuptake inhibitor.[21] (MAO stands for monoamine oxidase, which is a substance in the brain that breaks down neurotransmitters. By inhibiting MAO one increases neurotransmitter levels in the brain. Reuptake inhibition, which prevents neurotransmitters from returning into the terminal of the axon from which they were released, also increase neurotransmitter activity in the brain.) This means that resveratrol may have some antidepressant effects, as well as life extension properties, and that caution should be exercised in taking higher doses (over forty milligrams per day), as too high of a dose can make some people feel uncomfortably stimulated.

Pueraria Mirifica

Pueraria mirifica—known as Kwao Krua in Thailand—is a plant species found in Thailand and extends to a small area in Burma. The plant's underground tubers contain a number of chemicals called phytoestrogens, which are natural compounds that are very similar to a female sex hormone estriol.[22] *Pueraria mirifica* has been used as a breast enhancement supplement, as studies conducted by Thai and Japanese researchers have confirmed that Pueraria mirifica therapy was able to enhance breast size in women.[23] Early studies in England found that the plant had a beneficial effect on the skin and hair, as well as menopause.[24]

Pueraria mirifica has long been used by indigenous people in Thailand as a traditional medicine to treat hormone imbalances and the effects of aging in women. The phytoestrogens in it have been shown to be beneficial in reducing menopausal symptoms in post-menopausal women and it may help to reduce the risk of cancer. A study presented at the Emory University School of Medicine by Sayan Sawatsri M.D. and colleagues demonstrated that *Pueraria mirifica* can help to promote cellular mechanisms that improve the survival rate of vulnerable neurons in people with Alzheimer's disease.[25] It may also help to improve bone density and is sometimes used as a treatment for younger women with hormonal and skin problems.

Pueraria mirifica has also been shown to have adaptogenic properties. Adaptogenic herbs are unique in their ability to help balance hormone levels, lower stress, and help the body to maintain optimal homeostasis.

Deprenyl

Deprenyl (selegiline hydrochloride) is a moderate-level stimulant and antidepressant that has been shown to improve memory,[26] protect the brain against cell damage,[27] alleviate depression,[28] heighten sexual desire,[29] and extend the maximum life span of laboratory animals.[30,31] This impressive substance is available by prescription in the U.S., and it is primarily prescribed to help people with Parkinson's disease, memory disorder problems, and sometimes depression.

However, a lot of healthy people also use deprenyl to improve their mental performance, and it is considered by many people to be a "cognitive enhancer", or a "smart drug," like some of the substances that we discussed in chapter 4. What I didn't mention in chapter 4 is that many people report that smart drugs often have sexually-enhancing "side-effects", and deprenyl has one of the leading reputations in this area. According to Ward Dean, M.D., a gerontologist that I spoke with in Pensacola, Florida, "anything that improves brain function is probably going to improve sexual functioning." This is because sexuality and health go hand-in-hand, and sexual vitality is a pretty good indicator of overall health.

Deprenyl is a selective inhibitor of the dopamine-destroying enzyme MAO in the brain, similar to resveratrol, only much more powerful and specific. Because deprenyl inhibits this destructive enzyme, levels of the excitatory neurotransmitter dopamine rise in the brain, which generally causes people to feel more pleasure and become more physiologically aroused.

Interestingly, unlike most other MAO inhibitor drugs (like the antidepressant Nardil®), there are usually no dietary restrictions necessary when one takes deprenyl (or resveratrol). When taken at moderate levels (under ten milligrams), deprenyl only inhibits the action of a specific type of MAO—MAO B—which doesn't interfere with the body's ability to metabolize the amino acid tyrosine, like a broad-spectrum MAO inhibitor does. This is why most other MAO inhibiting drugs carry the serious danger of triggering a hypertensive reaction if one eats tyrosine-rich foods, like cheese. Deprenyl has been described by researchers as working with great precision in this regard, and the physicians that I spoke with agreed that it is unusually safe.

Deprenyl is better than safe; this truly remarkable drug has also been shown to significantly increase the maximum life span of laboratory animals.[32,33] To fully appreciate how significant deprenyl's life extension potential is, one has to understand the difference between maximum life span and average life span, as I described earlier. The laboratory animals in the deprenyl studies showed a forty percent increase in maximum life span. This is the human equivalent of living to be a hundred fifty years old. Since deprenyl's primary effects work the same in all mammalian brains, it stands to reason that deprenyl's life extension effects are likely to carry over to humans, just as the mental benefits do. Many people have certainly verified that the increase in sex drive occurs in both humans and laboratory animals.

Melatonin

Melatonin is a hormone that plays an important role in regulating people's circadian rhythms or sleep-wake cycles. It is produced by the pineal gland—a gland about the size of a pea that is located in the center of the brain—from the amino acid L-tryptophan. L-tryptophan produces the inhibitory neurotransmitter serotonin, which is the precursor to melatonin. As the day grows darker, the pineal gland starts to release melatonin and this is partly why we get tired at night. Levels of melatonin are highest in the blood prior to bedtime.

Melatonin levels decline with age, and this is one of the reasons that people often have more difficulty sleeping as they get older. Taking melatonin supplements at night can help people to sleep better as they age and many people use melatonin to reduce the symptoms of jet-lag when they travel. Several studies report that melatonin taken before bedtime decreases the amount of time it takes to fall asleep in elderly individuals with insomnia and that it also improves sleep in healthy individuals.[34]

A number of studies have also shown that melatonin has a variety of other health benefits, including increasing the lifespan of laboratory animals.[35] It acts as a powerful antioxidant and supplements have been shown to improve mood,[36] strengthen the immune system,[37] and reduce free radicals in the body.[38] By strengthening the immune system, melatonin supplements help to improve the body's resistance to cancer and other diseases. Melatonin supplements also lower blood pressure, help to normalize cholesterol levels, and prolong sexual vitality.[39]

DHEA

DHEA (dehydroepiandrosterone) is a steroid, a type of hormone that is produced by the adrenal glands, as well as by the brain and skin. It is the most abundant steroid in the human body, and it is the precursor to all adrenal hormones, which start to decline in both men and women at around the age of twenty-five.

DHEA production declines with age in such a consistent linear fashion that one's blood level of the hormone is often used as a bio-marker for aging, and low levels of it raise the risk of heart disease.[40] Since the body converts DHEA into all the other adrenal hormones, when DHEA levels begin to decline, so do the levels of these other hormones. This includes testosterone and estrogen, which are linked to both sex drive and performance.

When I interviewed the late Dr. William Regelson—who was a specialist in medical oncology at the Medical College of Virginia—he told me that by restoring one's DHEA levels to their youthful equivalent, an aging person can improve their memory, rejuvenate their immune system, increase their overall physical energy, reduce body fat, prevent heart disease, and enhance their libido.

According to Dr. Regelson, taking DHEA supplements can significantly increase sex drive, and he told me that "just about every adult age forty-five or older can benefit from taking DHEA." Dr. Regelson said that one of the most common comments that he heard from patients (as well as from colleagues and friends) who are taking DHEA is that it has renewed their interest in sex. Men in particular report this effect from taking DHEA.

According to the Massachusetts Male Aging Study, which investigated sexual function and activity in men aged forty to seventy, the incidence of impotency increased as DHEA levels declined.[41] Interestingly, many older men not only report an increased sex drive after they begin taking DHEA supplements, but also less of a problem achieving erection. In fact, many older men who have not had morning erections for years report that they suddenly began to experience them after taking DHEA.

DHEA is converted into testosterone, which is known to enhance libido in both men and women. This helps to explain why so many people report heightened sexual desire after they begin taking DHEA supplements. But there may be more to DHEA's enhancement of sexual desire and performance than simply raising testosterone levels. Because taking DHEA raises the levels of all adrenal hormones, it tends to make people feel more energetic, enhances feelings of well-being in general, and tends to improve overall heath.

DHEA is also thought to be a precursor to pheromones—invisible, airborne chemical messengers that travel between people, and often trigger sexual feelings. Taking DHEA supplements may help to boost pheromone production. This means that raising your DHEA levels may not only make you feel younger and healthier, it may also increase your level of sexual attractiveness as well.

Growth Hormone

Growth hormone (GH) is a hormone produced by the pituitary gland in the center of the brain, which stimulates cell reproduction and growth. Secretion levels of GH are highest during puberty—where they spur bodily growth—and they decline as people age or become obese. About a third of the population that is over the age of sixty isn't producing any measurable GH at all.

GH has a variety of important functions in the body. It repairs damaged tissue and promotes cell regeneration in the bones, vital organs and muscles. It is responsible for enhancing muscle growth, burning fat, and maintaining the immune system. GH also helps to support healthy blood pressure and cholesterol levels, and it reduces levels of C-reactive protein (CRP)—a protein produced by the liver that increases during systemic inflammation. Testing CRP levels in the blood is a useful way of assessing cardiovascular disease risk, as elevated CRP levels are correlated with a higher incidence of coronary artery disease.

In 1990, Daniel Rudman and his colleagues published a landmark study in the *New England Journal of Medicine* which looked at the effects of GH on twelve men who were over the age of sixty.[42] The twelve men were given GH injections three times a week for six months and were compared with nine men who received no treatment. The treatment resulted in a decrease in fatty tissue and increases in muscle mass and lumbar spine density. At the conclusion of the study all the men showed statistically significant increases in lean body mass and bone mineral density, while the control group did not. The authors of the study noted that the changes which they observed were the physiological equivalent of reversing the effects that would naturally develop over a ten to twenty year aging period.

More recently, in 2007, a Stanford University School of Medicine survey of clinical studies showed that the application of GH on healthy elderly patients increased muscle mass by two kilograms and decreased body fat by the same amount.[43] Because of these dramatic rejuvenating effects, many people have come to use GH as an effective anti-aging treatment. However, GH is destroyed by acids in the stomach so it needs to be taken by intramuscular injection, which many people find inconvenient, and there is a possibility of some side-effects—such as a thickening of bones and decreased thyroid output. Also, GH supplementation may be dangerous for people with cancer, or who are especially cancer-prone, as it significantly increases the growth rate of cancer cells.

However, in addition to injecting GH, there are some natural ways to increase GH production in the body. Some ways to stimulate GH production include exercise, dietary protein, maintaining low blood-sugar levels, and getting adequate amounts of sleep. There are also substances known as growth hormone releasers, but there is some controversy around how well they actually work. Oral GH releasers—such as amino acids like L-Arginine and L-Lysine—are generally not as powerful as taking GH by injection, and when people use these substances it may take longer for them to notice the desired effect. The amino acid L-Arginine has been shown to be the most effective amino acid for inducing GH release, but large amounts of it need to be taken, which can cause gastrointestinal disturbances.

However, a study published in 1981 by Dr. A. Isidori and colleagues demonstrated that a special form of the amino acid L-arginine called "arginine pyroglutamate," when used in combination with the amino acid L-lysine, can induce a significant amount of GH release when taken orally in relatively small amounts.[44] The results of this specific combination were quite impressive, causing a large GH release that was sustained for several hours.

Resveratrol, *pueraria mirifica*, and bioidentical hormone replacement therapy appear to significantly slow down the aging process, and these substances all work synergistically with EDTA chelation therapy. Heavy metal cleansing, pathogen-reducing, free radical quenching, and mitochondrial stimulation properties make EDTA an important antiaging medicine. It really does seem to offer genuine protection against some of the symptoms of aging and many people simply report that they look and feel younger after starting EDTA chelation therapy—especially when using it in combination with the other anti-aging supplements discussed in this chapter.

Currently, we have some extremely effective anti-aging tools at our disposal and better ones will be along soon. Doing all we can to help prevent aging at this particular moment in time is particularly important because the really big medical breakthroughs are coming along soon—and I suspect that you'd like to be around to benefit from them.

The Technology of Immortality

The field of biotechnology is rapidly advancing and practical stem cell therapies are getting closer every day. We stand on the brink of medicine's golden age. When I interviewed computer scientist and inventor Ray Kurzweil, he told me that he thought biotechnology, nanotechnology, artificial intelligence, and robotics will eventually allow people to live for indefinite periods of time without aging.

Dr. Kurzweil thinks that "nanobots, blood cell-size devices that could go inside the body and keep us healthy from inside" will be available in about two decades. So, Dr. Kurzweil believes, if we can just stay alive for another fifteen or twenty years we'll be able to, virtually, live forever. (It's important to note that Dr. Kurzweil has a very impressive track record as a technology forecaster—he received the 1999 National Medal of Technology, the nation's highest honor in technology, from President Clinton in a White House ceremony, and has received twelve honorary Doctorates and honors from three U.S. presidents.)

Perhaps the most compelling reason why radical life extension—as Dr. Kurzweil envisions—is possible is because not all animals age like we do. In fact, it appears that some animals don't age at all. Rockfish are routinely caught off the coast of Alaska that are hundreds of years old and are healthy and fertile. Whales have been known to live for over two hundred years without showing any signs of aging. A male whale that was over a hundred years old was harpooned while it was in the midst of having sex with a younger female. By studying these types of animals we can learn why they live so long without losing vitality or fertility and then apply that knowledge to extending the life span of human beings. In a future book, Dr. Gordon and I will explore the frontiers of anti-aging medicine.

If we would like to be around to participate in the great life extension breakthroughs that await us in the not-too-distant future then we need to take advantage of every tool that we have available to us to help improve our health and slow down the aging process. Because our world has become so polluted, and because our bodies are so loaded with toxins and pathogens, EDTA chelation therapy is absolutely essential for every person on this planet. Dr. Gordon even recommends that pets and farm animals be put on EDTA chelation therapy. But EDTA is not the only safe and effective heavy metal chelator that we have in our arsenal. In the next chapter we'll be discussing other safe and effective heavy metal chelators and different forms of chelation therapy.

Chapter 6

OTHER CHELATING AGENTS

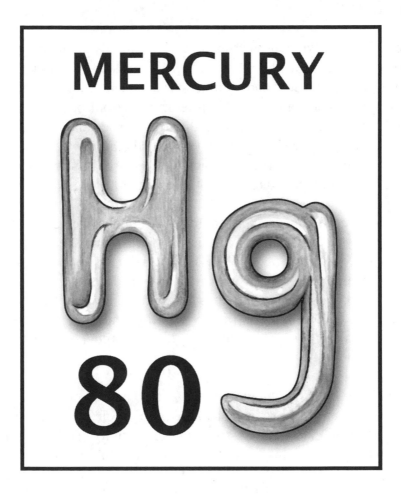

There are a number of other safe and effective chelating agents besides EDTA that can be used to help remove dangerous toxins and pathogens from the body. Some of these chelating agents are natural compounds, such as malic acid, alpha-lipoic acid, curcumin, garlic, vitamin C, and dimercaptosuccinic acid (DMSA). In this chapter we will discuss how these natural chelating agents work—and how they work synergistically together—to help remove toxic heavy metals from the body. We will also look at a powerful pharmaceutical chelating agent known as dimercapto-propane sulfonate (DMPS), as well as the necessary role that dietary fiber plays in helping to eliminate toxins from the body. Let's start by taking a look at malic acid.

Malic Acid

Malic acid—also known as fruit or apple acid—is abundantly found in many fruits and plants. Chemically, this organic acid is known as hydroxybutanedioic acid and hydroxysuccinic acid. Malic acid is tart to the taste and it plays a role in the taste of many sour or tart foods. For example, apples contain a lot of malic acid—especially green apples, which is why they tend to taste sour—and the amount of malic acid decreases as the fruit ripens. Malic acid is the source of tartness in many candies, such as SweeTarts® and Jolly Ranchers®.

This tart-tasting, organic acid is also found in animals, including humans, where it plays a key role in what is known as "the Krebs cycle"—a biochemical cycle that takes place inside the cells' mitochondria and produces energy in the form of ATP. Malic acid also has an oxygen-sparing effect. This means that it has the ability to lower cellular oxygen consumption without affecting its availability, and there are a number of indications that this is critical in controlling mitochondrial function in our cells.

A metabolite of malic acid—malate—is a source of energy from the Krebs cycle and it is the only metabolite of the cycle whose levels drop in concentration during exhaustive physical activity. The depletion of malate has also been linked to physical exhaustion, and this suggests that malic acid supplements can be used to help boost energy production. Your body manufactures malic acid, and, normally, when playing a role in the energy-producing Krebs cycle, it gets recycled again and again. However, if you're doing sustained aerobic exercise or strenuous physical activity you need to be able to produce more of it, and you may not be able to make as much malic acid as you need fast enough to meet the higher metabolic demand. This is one of the reasons why you may want to consider taking malic acid as a dietary supplement.

There is also some evidence that taking malic acid as a supplement, in combination with magnesium, may be helpful in treating some forms of fibromyalgia.[1] In a clinical study with fifteen fibromyalgia patients, a total daily dosage of 1,200-2,400 milligrams of malic acid was given, along with 300-600 mg of magnesium for eight weeks. (The magnesium was given because it is also necessary for ATP production and has oxygen-sparing effects.) All of the patients in the study reported a significant reduction in muscular pain within forty-eight hours of starting the supplement.

However, another study using just 1,200 milligrams of malic acid and 300 mg of magnesium failed to show a reduction in symptoms,[2] so there is some evidence that malic acid at higher doses—2,400 milligrams per day and magnesium at 600 milligrams per day—may be needed to treat the symptoms of fibromyalgia.

Besides playing a vital role in the Krebs cycle, malic acid also performs many other vital functions in the body—including the maintenance of proper acid balance and the removal of toxic metals by chelation. Malic acid is a powerful chelating agent. Malic acid has been found to be especially helpful in removing aluminum, and helps to remove lead, strontium, and other toxic heavy metals from the body.[3]

In a study at the University of Barcelona, toxicologists administered malic acid to mice exposed to aluminum at about one quarter of the dosage level that would kill approximately fifty percent of the animals.[4] Compared to other chelators, malic acid was shown to be the most effective at reducing aluminum toxicity—comparable with the synthetic chelator deferoxamine mesylate, without any of the side effects. Studies suggest that a dosage of around two thousand milligrams of malic acid per day would be consistent with the dosages that were shown to produce beneficial results under laboratory conditions. An apple generally contains several hundred milligrams of malic acid, so it may take more than just an apple a day to keep the doctor away. Although it is possible to consume the two thousand milligram per day suggested dosage entirely from apples, it is far easier to simply take malic acid in supplement form.

Alpha-Lipoic Acid

Alpha-lipoic acid (ALA) is a fat-soluble, sulfur-containing enzyme, which operates as a cofactor in the metabolism of glucose and oxygen utilization. It also plays a crucial role in the mitochondrial production of energy in the body. ALA is a coenzyme in the metabolic process necessary for the conversion of glucose to ATP (energy). Soon after its discovery in 1950, ALA was shown to provide effective protection against toxin and radiation damage. It is now recognized as a powerful antioxidant and chelating agent.[5] ALA has a strong ability to disarm oxygen free radicals and a high affinity for chelating undesirable ionized metals that can generate free radicals. It also has anti-glycation capabilities, and—unlike other antioxidants—is active as a free radical scavenger in both its fat-soluble and water-soluble phases.

In the past fifty-seven years there have been over eight hundred research papers published on ALA and new discoveries continue to evolve. When I interviewed U.C. Berkeley researcher, Dr. Lester Packer, he referred to ALA as the "ideal antioxidant," not only because it works as a powerful antioxidant on its own, but also because it acts in a synergistic fashion with other antioxidants.

As an antioxidant, ALA is unique for a number of reasons. It is both fat and water soluble, which means that ALA is easily absorbed and transported across cell membranes, offering us protection against free radical damage both inside and outside the cells in our body. This is unlike other antioxidants which only provide extra cellular protection. The structure of ALA is very small, and this also allows it to easily slip through cell membranes. Many other antioxidants are too large to pass through the cell membrane. So ALA slips in and out of cells very easily, where it acts as a powerful free radical scavenger. However, its claim to fame as the "ideal antioxidant" resides in its ability to recycle and rejuvenate other antioxidants.

ALA works to recycle and reactivate free radical scavengers obtained from our diet—such as vitamins C and E—thereby maximizing utilization of these vitamins as antioxidants. ALA has the same effect on endogenously-produced (within the body) antioxidants, such as thioredoxin and glutathione. Even after these vitamins and endogenously-produced antioxidants have already been oxidized, ALA can reactivate them. So if you are not getting enough vitamin C or E in your diet, ALA supplements can help compensate for the difference.

Another property that makes ALA an unusually effective antioxidant is that it possesses antioxidant properties in both its original form as well as its reduced form (known as dihydrolipoic acid or DHLA). In fact, DHLA is an even more potent antioxidant than ALA. Most antioxidant substances, like vitamins C and E, only act as antioxidants in their reduced forms. After they have donated an electron, they are then incapacitated as an antioxidant unless they are regenerated by another antioxidant like ALA.

Although ALA was originally thought to be a vitamin, most researchers now believe that the liver synthesizes it in small amounts. However, due to the way ALA functions synergistically with certain vitamins (the antioxidant B vitamins, vitamin C, and vitamin E), some researchers suspect that it still might be an essential nutrient. But even though ALA's entire metabolic pathway in the body is not clearly understood, researchers agree that levels of this important enzyme decrease with age, and with that decline many of the body's rejuvenating abilities are lost.

In addition to its rejuvenating antioxidant abilities, ALA also helps to prevent glycation damage—which results from blood-sugar levels that are too high—and this is why it can be helpful in treating diabetes. ALA has been used throughout Europe to control high blood sugar levels, as well as for the prevention and treatment of diabetic complications, such as neuropathy, atherosclerosis, and renal disease. ALA appears to be the most potent natural insulin mimicker known; it works even better than Vanadyl sulfate and Chromium.

ALA also helps to prevent the generalized glycation damage that everyone experiences from simply metabolizing sugar, which results in dangerous cross-linked proteins throughout the body, and is the source of much of what we perceive as aging—a loss of skin elasticity, stiffening of the arteries, cataracts, age spots, etc. ALA has been shown to prevent cataracts, and it reduces the risk of age-related macular degeneration and other symptoms of aging.[6] There is evidence that ALA helps to slow down numerous aspects of the aging process, through its anti-glycation abilities, and by protecting the brain, and by preserving intracellular mitochondria (which supply the basic energy that regulates every cell in the body).[7]

ALA supplementation has been shown to be beneficial in helping to treat a variety of medical problems besides diabetes and the formation of cataracts. It is also especially useful in the treatment of neurodegenerative disorders and in the prevention of cardiovascular disease. ALA can help to lower elevated cholesterol levels and this makes it a great protector against atherosclerosis (the condition which underlies cardiovascular disease). A study done with mice found that supplements of lipoic acid can inhibit formation of arterial lesions, lower triglycerides, and reduce blood vessel inflammation and weight gain—all key factors for addressing cardiovascular disease.[8]

Free radicals negatively modify LDL (low density lipoprotein) cholesterol, which is one of the primary contributors to the undesirable cholesterol deposits which form atherosclerotic plaques in the blood vessels. Sufficient levels of vitamin E can protect against this type of free radical damage, and since ALA extends the life of vitamin E, it also increases protection from this type of damage.[9]

ALA can also help to retard the activation of the HIV virus[10] (which is believed to cause AIDS), and it can be used a treatment for AIDS. Several important research findings indicate that ALA may offer some hope for those who suffer from AIDS. Research reveals that HIV patients have low levels of a potent endogenous (from within the body) antioxidant called glutathione. Glutathione is an important antioxidant that is utilized within cells and it is a major repair enzyme. One study demonstrated that when ALA is administered to the body's T cells (cells involved in immune protection), there is a dramatic rise in intracellular glutathione levels.[11]

Another study found that ALA has a buffering effect on detrimental gene activation, a process which is induced by the rampage of free radicals. Expression of HIV is dependent upon aberrant gene activation. In several studies ALA and other antioxidants were effective in inhibiting the activation of this mechanism.[12] Because of these findings, researchers have proposed using ALA as a therapeutic adjunct to treating HIV infection.

ALA may help to prevent brain damage when the brain is deprived of oxygen due to stroke or cardiac arrest. Damage to the brain commonly occurs during these situations because of the combination of ischemia (lack of oxygen) and reperfusion (rapid reoxygenation). Most of the brain damage usually occurs during reperfusion, which is primarily attributed to injury from oxygen free radicals. When experimental animals are treated with ALA before being exposed to both ischemia and reperfusion, there is a significant reduction of brain damage.[13]

ALA may also help with age-related memory decline. It has the potential for enhancing or preserving cognitive abilities, protecting against Parkinson's disease, and helping to slow down the progression of Alzheimer's disease. In one experiment with mice, ALA demonstrated an improvement in the long-term memory of older mice, after being administered for a period of fifteen days.[14] However, there was no change among the younger mice. It appears that ALA alleviated certain neurotransmitter (NMDA) receptor deficits in the older animals.

There is reason to believe that ALA and other antioxidants may also be helpful in preventing cancer,[15] since free radical damage to DNA is thought to be a main factor in causing cells to become cancerous. ALA can revive and rejuvenate other antioxidant substrates present in the body,[16] like the spent ascorbate and tocopherol radicals produced when vitamin C and vitamin E disarm higher-energy free radicals.

ALA has also been shown to chelate heavy metals.[17] It is most effective at chelating copper, lead, and mercury. This mighty, multipurpose enzyme is a powerful enough chelator that it can actually be used to chelate mercury in cases of mercury poisoning, although it is rarely used as a first-line treatment for this (due, partially, to conventional medicine's reliance upon pharmaceutical rather than nutritional agents, and, possibly, because of the greater clinical effectiveness of the chelating agents dimercaptosuccinic acid (DMSA) and dimercapto-propane sulfonate (DMPS), which we will discuss in the following sections of this chapter). Actually, ALA is unusually suited for the purpose of chelating mercury poisoning because it can penetrate both the blood-brain barrier and the cell membrane. ALA is an extremely important heavy metal chelator because—as we've repeated numerous times throughout this book—everyone is suffering from some degree of mercury poisoning.

There are a growing number of studies substantiating the multiple benefits of ALA and showing that doses of six hundred to a thousand milligrams a day produce the greatest health benefits for health maintenance and preventive purposes. ALA can be obtained from the diet, and spinach is an especially rich source. However, it would be very difficult to obtain the levels of ALA necessary to provide the health benefits shown in studies from diet alone, so supplementation is suggested.

Curcumin

Curcumin and other "curcuminoids" are a class of polyphenols with extraordinary health-enhancing properties. Curcumin is derived from the Indian spice turmeric, which is a member of the ginger family. Turmeric was originally valued in Southeast Asia because of its ability to maintain the freshness of food and is commonly used in curry as a spice. Along with the other curcuminoids—such as demethoxycurcumin, bisdemethoxycurcumin, and cyclocurcumin—it has a yellow pigment and is not very soluble in water. Turmeric extract is composed of around three to five percent curcuminoids, and it has long been used in Ayurvedic medicine to treat a variety of ailments—such as liver disease and problems with the urinary tract. In recent years, there has been a large amount of research done on curcumin and other curcuminoids.

Studies have shown that curcumin has powerful anti-inflammatory and antioxidant properties, which make it helpful in preventing a wide range of disorders. Some studies show that curcumin's anti-inflammatory properties may be due to its ability to inhibit the biosynthesis of intercellular messengers known as eicosanoids, which can lead to silent inflammation.[18] Curcumin and other components of turmeric have been shown to help prevent and treat cancer,[19, 20, 21] to be helpful in treating AIDS,[22] and possibly as a treatment for cystic fibrosis.[23] It is also thought to help prevent Alzheimer's disease for a number of reasons.[24]

Curcumin has also been shown to have powerful anti-amyloid properties, and this is one of the primary reasons why it is thought to be a powerful preventer of Alzheimer's disease.[25] Amyloids are complex proteins that are deposited in various tissues and these protein deposits—or plaque— are associated with certain diseases. Although it is unclear whether these amyloid deposits are the cause of, or a sign of, a particular disease, there is clearly a correlation between the two.

In Alzheimer's disease deposits of a special type of amyloid known as "beta-amyloid protein" are found in the brain. In other illnesses the deposits of amyloid may be localized in particular diseased organs, such as in the pancreas with type 2 diabetes. Amyloid may also be deposited widely throughout the body, as in a condition known as "systemic amyloidosis." Curcumin has been shown to help prevent amyloid from being deposited into tissues throughout the body, so it may be helpful in preventing or treating these conditions.

A study done at UCLA in 2004 showed that curcumin might inhibit the accumulation of destructive beta-amyloid in the brains of Alzheimer's disease patients and also break up existing plaques associated with the disease. Further evidence that curcumin may be helpful in the prevention of Alzheimer's disease comes from epidemiological studies done in India—a country where turmeric consumption is widespread—which show that it has one of the lowest prevalence rates of Alzheimer's disease in the world.

There is also evidence that curcumin helps to prevent certain types of cancer. Curcumin acts as a free radical scavenger, which inhibits lipid peroxidation and oxidative DNA damage, and helps to protect against cancer. It also has anticancer effects that stem from its ability to induce apoptosis (cellular suicide) in cancer cells without toxic effects on healthy cells. Studies show that when curcumin is added to the diet given to rats or mice previously given a carcinogen, it significantly reduces colon carcinogenesis,[26] and another study indicates that curcumin may suppress a cancer-causing gene involved in mechanisms of malignant tumor formation.[27]

Curcumin is also a heavy metal chelator. It removes lead, iron, and other metals from the body and a recent study done by Dairam, Limson, and colleagues showed that it significantly reduces lead-induced memory deficits in laboratory animals.[28] Studies show that curcumin helps to reverse lead neurotoxity and it has also been shown to have a neuroprotective effect.[29]

In addition to helping to prevent Alzheimer's disease, curcumin may help to improve cognitive functioning in general. A survey of over a thousand Asians—between the ages of 60 and 93—who ate yellow curry sauce once every six months or more demonstrated superior cognitive performance compared with those who did not.[30] However, this effect may actually be due to curcumin's ability to chelate heavy metals from the body, as it could simply be removing possible lead-induced memory deficits created by environmental toxins. Or it could be that people who ate curry tended to have healthier habits in general. Or there could be some completely different relationship, so more research in this area is needed.

I suspect that further research into curcumin and other curcuminoids will reveal a bounty of health-enhancing treasures. As a personal side note, I'd like to add that I take curcumin several times daily largely because of it's ability to enhance my sexual performance, as it substantially increases the strength of my orgasms. I haven't read about this interesting effect elsewhere, but I was certainly happy to discover that preventing cancer, Alzheimer's disease, and other inflammatory-based diseases can be so much fun.

Garlic, Vitamin C, and Dietary Fiber

In chapter 2 we learned about garlic's antibiotic abilities, vitamin C's antioxidant properties, and the many health benefits that come from obtaining an adequate amount of dietary fiber in one's diet. Garlic, vitamin C, and dietary fiber are also effective chelating agents.

Studies show that garlic will chelate lead and mercury, as well as other heavy metals and toxins.[31] According to Dr. Gordon, "even red dye # 40 will be chelated out by garlic." In addition to its well-established antibiotic properties (which we discussed in chapter 2), some studies also show that garlic may have the potential to lower cholesterol levels[32] and reduce the risk of cardiovascular disease. [33, 34]

So garlic not only helps to chelate heavy metals from the body and remove toxins, it also helps to prevent the damage caused by dangerous metals and provides numerous other health benefits. The same is true for vitamin C and dietary fiber. Vitamin C has been shown to help chelate heavy metals from the body and to reduce the harmful effects of lead, aluminum, copper, silica, and radiation due to its powerful antioxidant properties.[35] Preliminary studies with vitamin C report that dosages of three thousand milligrams a day help to remove aluminum from brain cells, which has important implications for helping to prevent Alzheimer's disease and other neurological disorders.

Dietary fiber is also an effective heavy metal chelator and it helps to remove all sorts of toxins from the body. In fact, fiber is such a strong chelator that too much unleavened bread can even induce a zinc deficiency. Garlic, vitamin C and dietary fiber are three of the most important natural chelating agents and they should be a part of everyone's daily regime. Another important—but less well-known—natural chelator is a substance known as DMSA.

DMSA

Dimercaptosuccinic acid (DMSA) is a powerful, water-soluble chelating agent that has been used for removing heavy metals from the body since the 1950s. This safe and effective chelating agent is marketed under the trade name Chemet® in the U.S.—with all sorts of additives and preservatives, my coauthor points out—although it is actually a valuable source of succinic acid, an important nutrient. Like malic acid, succinic acid is a necessary part of "the Krebs cycle"—a biochemical cycle that takes place inside the cells' mitochondria and produces energy in the form of ATP.

DMSA is the only chelating agent that is considered to be as effective when taken orally as when it is given through an I.V. route. It binds to arsenic, aluminum, mercury, lead, and other heavy metals and carries them out of the body through the kidneys. DMSA is approved by the FDA for removing lead and mercury from the brains of children who are suffering from lead or mercury poisoning, as this unusually effective chelating agent is capable of crossing the blood/brain barrier. It is currently the only approved oral medication in the U.S. for children with high levels of lead or mercury, although—because our environment has become so toxic with heavy metals—my coauthor believes that it has many more applications. This is because DMSA is such an effective chelator and, like EDTA, it is safe and relatively nontoxic.

Although DMSA has an excellent track record of being both safe and effective, an internet search on DMSA will reveal that a number of people think that using DMSA chelation therapy carries an elevated risk for a certain segment of the population—pregnant mothers and people with mercury amalgam dental fillings. My coauthor thinks that both of these risks have been greatly exaggerated, and that the benefits of having less lead and mercury in an adult brain or in that of a growing fetus are well documented. Dr. Gordon points out that every choice we make involves potential benefits and risks. After reviewing all of the documented benefits that result from using effective chelators and lowering the levels of toxic metals in the body, Dr. Gordon concludes that the documented benefits far outweigh the potential risks associated with using effective chelators such as DMSA or EDTA regularly, at least for a few months every year.

A study done at Cornell University on pregnant rats showed some evidence suggesting that DMSA could have problematic side-effects for the developing mammalian immune system.[36] However, this same study also showed that DMSA actually reversed several harmful effects of lead exposure, such as altered body weight and spleen weight in rat pups. It also increased levels of tumor necrosis factor (TNF) and interleukin-4 (IL-4). TNF has been shown to exhibit antiproliferative effects against a wide variety of tumor cell lines, and interleukin-4 is a protein that stimulates the immune system to develop new cells.

There are also a number of warnings on the internet cautioning people with mercury amalgam dental fillings against practicing DMSA chelation therapy because they believe that there is a danger that DMSA can bind to the mercury in one's mouth and then carry it into the brain and nervous system—although, my coauthor states, there is little evidence that this happens. These warnings suggest that people have their mercury dental fillings removed and replaced with nontoxic dental fillings before beginning DMSA chelation therapy.

While my coauthor agrees that removing mercury amalgam dental fillings is certainly a good idea, he actually thinks that just the opposite is true. Dr. Gordon thinks that those unfortunate folks with toxic mercury amalgam fillings in their mouth should be using DMSA and/or EDTA to help remove the mercury that is coming from their teeth every time they chew. Studies show that in a tooth with mercury amalgam dental fillings the process of chewing will release toxic mercury vapors for many years. DMSA binds to this mercury and carries it out of the body. (Dr. Gordon has also formulated a EDTA-based chewing gum, to be used by people with mercury amalgam dental fillings after a meal, which helps to chelate the mercury that has been released.)

Some people believe that a number of cases of multiple sclerosis (MS)— a disease of the nervous system in which the fatty insulating tissue around nerve fibers begins to degrade—are aggravated by dental mercury in the nervous system, and there is some evidence to support this claim. DMSA is capable of crossing the blood/brain barrier and carrying mercury out of the brain and some MS patients have reported favorable changes in their quality of life once they started DMSA chelation therapy.

DMSA is considered to be much safer than DMPS (Dimercapto-1-propane sulfonate), another powerful chelator, which we will discuss in the next section. Research has shown that DMSA is around three times less toxic than DMPS. DMSA also works well with other chelators. A study published in 1994 by Drs. Tandon and Singh showed that the administration of EDTA or DMSA was more effective than that of DMPS.[37] It also showed that the combination of EDTA and DMSA was more efficient than that of EDTA and DMPS, or the individual chelators, in enhancing the excretion of lead from the body, and in restoring lead-induced inhibition of a variety of blood factors.

A number of other studies also show synergistic effects from combining DMSA and EDTA. "However," according to Dr. Gordon's colleague Dr. Jerry Schlesser, "in certain situations it is not always the ideal way to chelate, because in some cases combining them actually slightly lowers the effective urinary excretion." Nevertheless, Dr. Gordon points out that "the definitive studies on fecal and/or total excretion have not been done. Since chelators are always enhancing the excretion of toxic metals from your body, there will always be benefits—but the final decision regarding the use of combinations of chelators in a given patient should be based upon the clinical picture and laboratory findings on an individual basis. For general detoxification purposes, the combined use of DMSA and EDTA makes sense, but not always. That's why we don't put EDTA and DMSA together in our formulations."

In a study by Juresa, Blanusa, and colleagues, DMSA and DMPS were tested for their efficiency in mercury removal in the presence and in the absence of the essential mineral selenium.[38] The study showed that inorganic selenium (as sodium selenite) decreases the efficiency of DMSA and DMPS in mercury removal from the body. This suggests that it may be optimal to take DMSA and selenium several hours apart. However, most minerals, like copper and zinc or calcium and magnesium are also somewhat better absorbed if taken separately, and for many people this may not always be convenient and practical. Because of this, and because Dr. Gordon is convinced that most people will benefit greatly from increased selenium intake to help counteract the toxic metals in their bodies, he routinely has his patients take selenium and their chelators at the same time, even though there could be some slight advantage to separating them.

The inconvenience of having to take selenium and DMSA several hours apart leads to a strong potential for less compliance. So Dr. Gordon, who is aware of these studies, routinely combines his selenium with his chelators, and generally takes his DMSA with his EDTA. Dr. Gordon believes that our current intake of selenium is far too low to deal with our heavy metal exposures, and he often recommends aggressive selenium supplementation. When patients are under the care of a health professional who monitors their blood-selenium levels, using a competent lab (such as Doctor's Data) so as to avoid the potential of selenium toxicity, Dr. Gordon often recommends dosages of four hundred to eight hundred micrograms per day. This is because selenium has been shown to be very effective in helping offset the toxicity of mercury and lead.

Dr. Gordon thinks that any minimal improvement that might be accomplished by taking DMSA and selenium separately will—for most people—be lost by the inconvenience of having to do so. However, Dr. Gordon also points out that this particular study was done with an inorganic form of selenium known as selenium selenite. In his formulas he uses an organic amino acid complex form of selenium, such as "methyl-selenocysteine," which is not the same as the inorganic form of selenium that DMSA binds to.

In addition to effectively removing toxic heavy metals from the body, and binding to selenium, DMSA chelation therapy, like EDTA chelation therapy, also removes essential minerals—such as calcium, magnesium, potassium, and zinc—so it is important to always take a highly absorbable multi mineral supplement after taking DMSA.

DMPS

Dimercapto-1-propane sulfonate (DMPS) is a powerful, tissue permeable metal chelator. It was developed in the Soviet Union in 1958 and is currently a registered drug in Germany. Consecutive DMPS injections have been shown to significantly decrease total mercury concentrations in the kidney, brain, and blood. DMPS has been found to be a highly effective chelating agent, particularly with respect to promoting mercury elimination following mercury exposure. The efficacy of DMPS as a mercury chelator appears to be related to consecutive administration in consistent dosages, rather than to the magnitude of the dose received.

DMPS has been used extensively in Europe and on a limited basis in North America as a treatment for mercury, arsenic, or lead intoxication. In addition to being used as a metal chelator, DMPS is also sometimes used as a diagnostic tool to approximate mercury body burden. Resting urine or blood levels of mercury bear little relationship to body burden of mercury in cases of long standing, low level intoxication, such as that which may occur from mercury dental amalgams. Because DMPS permeates the tissue and carries it out of the body, it can help to give a more accurate approximation of how much mercury there actually is in one's body.

However, DMPS is not nearly as safe as the other chelators that we've discussed in this book. DMPS is not approved by the FDA and it is considered an experimental drug in the U.S. Some people do not tolerate DMPS well. This is especially true for those who have damage in the central nervous system, such as those with MS or children with fragile brain architecture. DMPS is also sometimes associated with serious side effects, such as severe gastrointestinal disturbances and cognitive dysfunctions. In fact, an upset patient started a Web site called DMPS Backfire to collect information from people who have had adverse effects from this drug, because she believes that her "life was derailed by a single injection of DMPS." She reports symptoms that include "gnawing stomach pains, diarrhea, nausea, dizziness, relentless headache, exhaustion, chest pains, numbness in my extremities, and other symptoms."

Because of these sometimes serious side-effects my coauthor says that he "shys away" from using DMPS as a chelating agent. Dr. Gordon finds these side-effects puzzling, as this appears to be a recent phenomena. According to Dr. Gordon, the DMPS that he used to get from Moscow thirty years ago had significantly fewer side-effects than the DMPS that comes from Germany today and it seemed "as safe as water." Other researchers and physicians have noticed this increase in side-effects as well, and it may be traceable to different manufacturing processes, but no one seems to know for sure.

Also, as with DMSA, people with mercury amalgam dental fillings are warned against practicing DMPS chelation therapy because there is the danger that it can bind to the mercury in your mouth and carry it into the nervous system. So, as with DMSA, it is suggested that people have their mercury dental fillings removed and replaced with nontoxic dental fillings before beginning DMPS chelation therapy. DMPS chelation therapy, like EDTA and DMSA chelation therapy, also removes important minerals, so it is important to always take a highly absorbable multi-mineral supplement several hours after a DMPS treatment.

The Future of Chelation Therapy and Beyond

As we've learned in this book, chelation therapy should be a part of everyone's daily regime. In a future book, my coauthor and I will explore the potential of these other forms of chelation therapy—as well as other ways to improve health and extend life—in greater depth. In the years to come, new and even more effective forms of chelation therapy will surely be developed, and we look forward to these advances with great excitement. However, let us thank the stars that we already have a treasure trove of tools available to us that anyone can use to improve their health today.

We are living in truly astonishing times. Although our current healthcare system appears to be crumbling around us, we are simultaneously witnessing a rapidly-advancing biotechnology revolution that promises to forever change the course of human history. New possibilities are emerging everywhere we turn, and there is enormous cause for hope. When we look out onto the frontiers of medicine we see an incredible vista blossoming with possibilities that stagger the mind and border on the miraculous. New advances in medicine promise to help humanity end countless generations of suffering and deliver us into a golden age where disease and aging are merely subjects that we learn about in history class, and the boundaries of our physical capacities are limited only by our imaginations.

We hope that you found the suggestions in this book helpful. Chelation therapy and proper nutritional support can provide us with bridges to the awe-inspiring possibilities that the future holds in store, and they offer us the hope that we can all live longer, healthier, and happier lives right now.

APPENDIX A

ELATION OVER CHELATION:
AN INTERVIEW WITH DR. GARRY GORDON

BY DAVID JAY BROWN

To follow is an interview that I did with Dr. Gordon about heavy metal toxicity and chelation therapy. In the interview we spoke about the dangers of environmental toxins, the benefits of chelation therapy, the differences between oral and I.V. chelation therapies, how chelation therapy effects bone growth, and many other topics that are important for optimal health.

David: Can you tell me why you think that chelation therapy is important, and what the primary differences between oral EDTA chelation and intravenous chelation are?

Dr. Gordon: Chelation therapy is so important because—from the moment we're born—every man, woman, and child today has an average of a thousand times more lead in their bones than their ancestors. This is because the lead downloads from the mother. In fact, according to the latest research, the best way for a woman to get rid of lead in her body is to have a baby, because the lead goes into the baby. So, from the moment you're born, you have too much lead, mercury, and cadmium in your body. According to the *Archives of Internal Medicine*, these metals are now proven to have adverse effects on your morbidity and mortality. It's documented that the lower you keep your lead level throughout your life, the longer you live, and the less likely you are to get cancer, diabetes, hypertension, etc.

So everybody today needs chelation. This is because we have polluted our Earth. Today the planet has so much lead that even if you're raising grapes to make vinegar in Italy, the vinegar will have lead in it, because the soil has lead. There's no place to escape. Every leaf, every blade of grass, is now coated with particulate matter, which comes from the burning of fossil fuels like coal and is carried on the air. So, the oceans are loaded with mercury. There's nothing you can eat that doesn't have these dangerous heavy metals. So chelation is the only way you're going to have optimal health. These metals are poisons to the enzymes in your body that allow you to make the ten billion new cells you have to make every day, and the ability of our body to repair itself continuously is impeded when enzyme function is defeated.

So, to keep it really simple, the difference between I.V. and oral chelation is that oral chelation is a bit like washing your car. It's a good idea and it looks pretty good. I.V. is like doing a Simonize®. It does a deeper cleansing, but not everybody can afford to Simonize® their car. So everybody needs to be doing the oral chelation every day of their life. That way they'll be keeping their body as clean as they can. What we've done is we've taken the oral EDTA and mixed it with other natural products that happen to look and function in the body the same as heparin.

I have replaced Coumadin® in my patients and they don't die of blood clots. 1.4 million people in the United States die each year from what they call a heart attack or stroke, but it's really a blood clot. So, to me, oral chelation is absolutely the only way of assuring that my patients don't show up in an emergency room with fatal hearts or strokes. It's been twenty years now, and we have yet to hear of the first person having a fatal heart attack or stroke while taking the oral program that I devised. But the intravenous chelation is a deeper cleansing, so one doesn't replace the other.

The sad thing is that I was overly enthusiastic thirty years ago and I thought that the intravenous chelation was actually reversing obstructive plaque on our arteries, taking away arteriosclerosis. It turns out that in some people it can reverse plaque, but many people still had an eighty or ninety percent blockage in their vessels. However, many of these people still find that their memory or vision improves, their sex life gets better, their feet get warmer, their blood pressure grows more normal, and they can suddenly run upstairs.

The reasons that we've restored health to them is much more tied to the concept of nitric oxide acting as an endothelial relaxing factor, which enhances blood flow through capillaries. This actually turns out to be more important than taking the plaque out of your artery, because now you're profusing the tissue efficiently, and the lead inhibits nitric oxide synthases. Removing the lead improves the efficiency of nitric oxide, which helps to enhance blood flow and improve circulation. So pollution is one of the reasons that people have poor circulation.

Oral chelation does two things. It takes the lead out, and when it's in the proper formulas that are available today, it replaces Coumadin®, aspirin, or Plavix®, which has recently been shown to be dangerous. Natural products are safer, but, unfortunately, people have to pay for natural products. It's not going to be covered by their insurance. But we have the advantage that we don't do what Coumadin® does. Coumadin® helps to turn your blood vessel into bone. It actually is proven to do that. This means that you get hard blood vessels. Now, the harder your blood vessels become, the higher your blood pressure goes, and the sooner you're going to die of a complication from vascular disease.

So the need for chelation is universal. We have to make it affordable, and nothing is as convenient as oral chelation. The oral chelation can be as simple as EDTA, which is my favorite molecule. It's four molecules of vinegar, and it has never been shown to cause any damage when taken, as long as there is a reasonable intake of good minerals with it. This is because EDTA is not so clever that it binds only to lead, mercury, and cadmium. It will also take out zinc. So you could have the embarrassing situation of somebody taking a chelating agent, and not taking a good multiple that has zinc, and aggravating the zinc deficiency that much of the American population has. That would not be in their best interest.

So with chelation we do have to maintain a constant good mineral input, but that's important anyhow if you're going to be healthy. Everybody needs to know that most people are not getting enough selenium. They're not getting enough magnesium. Hardly anyone is getting enough vitamin D, enough vitamin B-6, enough vitamin C, etc. All these nutrients are not adequately present in our diets, so we have to supplement. After we have the supplements going in, then people need to be on oral chelation daily from as early as possible. This way, we'll have less infections in childhood. We'll have less death and longer life spans.

The intravenous chelation is really wonderful, because it's such a deep cleansing. People who put off doing something about their health for years sometimes walk in my office, and it looks like we're going to have to amputate their right foot, or they're going to have to be placed in an old folk's home, because they don't remember their last name anymore. Then the deep cleansing of intravenous chelation can do things that you simply couldn't do rapidly enough with oral chelation to get the patient out of their problem.

David: How does EDTA chelation therapy affect blood circulation and how can it be used to promote cardiovascular health?

Dr. Gordon: EDTA is essentially four molecules of vinegar and chelation is a natural process. The word "chelation" came from the Greek word "claw." Somebody suggested the metaphor that EDTA is like using a hamburger as an easy way to give your dog a pill, because you hide the pill in the protein. EDTA is essentially a man-made synthetic amino acid, which hides the lead, mercury, cadmium, or other metal inside of it, so that it is finally able to exit the body with a higher efficiency. Every human being on Earth today is breathing in tremendous amounts of lead, mercury, and cadmium because we burn coal in order to turn on the power plants and generate electricity around the world. Every time we turn on a power plant we create more cases of autism.

We're beginning to realize that the blood circulation in our bodies, and our cardiovascular health in general, is significantly impaired in obvious ways due to lead poisoning. We now know that every human being on Earth has an average of over one thousand times more lead in every tissue than we did in pre-industrial times. Of course most of the lead gets concentrated in certain tissues—like, for example, more in the bones than in the heart. But everybody on Earth has a minimum of about a thousand times more lead in their bones than in any human bones from over two hundred years. So we're reaching the point of maximum tolerance, with the net result being that as the bones are filled with lead and they can't handle any more, so it spills over and starts to accumulate in the heart, kidney, liver, and brain.

A year ago Debra Schaumberg at Harvard University published her important research in the *Journal of the American Medical Association*, showing that the higher the percentage of lead that there is in the bones the sooner people go blind from cataracts. This is why I think that everyone today needs to be on some kind of chelation therapy. You see, it's not just the heart that we're helping—it's the whole body. The kidneys are loaded with heavy metals that are impairing kidney function. Even the *New England Journal of Medicine* claimed about two years ago that if more people would receive calcium EDTA we might largely eliminate renal failure. In other words, there wouldn't be any people having to live on dialysis. So it's not just the heart we're helping. We're also protecting the bones and the rest of the body.

Nitric oxide is very important for proper cardiovascular health, and this is an important area that all doctors can relate to. Nitric oxide was the molecule of the year a few years ago. This is not the laughing gas that the dentist gives you; that's nitrous oxide. Nitric oxide is an extremely important molecule in our body that was previously called "endothelial relaxing factor." Endothelium is the Saran™ Wrap-like lining that is the inside lining of every blood vessel in your body, and if you can make good levels of nitric oxide, or endothelial relaxing factor, then you're going to have your blood vessels relaxed instead of constricted. And if they're relaxed then they're open and they let more blood go through.

The net result is that the person then has less angina, more ability to walk miles without getting leg cramps, better vision, and better memory. So throughout the whole body we assist everything when we use chelation therapy. But the way in which EDTA affects nitric oxide is only a tiny piece of the whole story, because we all have too much lead in our body. There is no escape. You can't move to the Arctic or the Antarctic. It's everywhere, and when it's in our bodies it is adversely affecting the tissue that the lead accumulates in. So we can state unequivocally that if your heart has too much lead in it then even the pumping function of your heart will be affected.

In fact, there's a disease called idiopathic dilated hypertrophic cardiomyopathy, where the heart muscle is enlarged, and when the tissue is analyzed it can have as much as a ten thousand-fold increase in the levels of mercury, lead, or cadmium. So now things are starting to come together. Thirty-five years ago no one dreamed that we would actually have levels of toxic metals like cadmium, lead, and mercury in the actual muscle of the heart.

We now know that the blood flow throughout your whole body—through your capillaries, arteries and veins—is also effected by the level of lead. When lead levels go up our body is unable to convert a certain amino acid into nitric oxide. When we eat a good meal we are getting an amino acid called arginine, and in a healthy body that isn't lead-toxic, that arginine can be converted to nitric oxide, which would then mean that all the blood vessels would be open and the person would have less angina, almost like a tablet we used for many years called nitroglycerin. A person could put nitroglycerin under their tongue and it would stop their chest from being locked in pain by relaxing vessels and letting things work. So cardiovascular health and chelation are absolutely mandatory, and that's keeping the story to the simple part of it. My work in chelation has gone to the more complex part of it, which is the blood-clotting part of the story.

The blood-clotting part of the story comes into play when we realize that almost one out of two people in America still die of heart attacks and strokes—and experts are pretty much agreeing today that well over eighty percent of heart attacks are, in the final analysis, truly due to a blood clot. This has caused a lot of people to get excited about trying to take aspirin—which we find largely worthless, and in fact dangerous. Aspirin is vastly oversold for its capabilities and it gives people a false sense of security. People think that if they're taking an aspirin that they are going to have less clots whereas thirty percent of people have no benefit whatsoever in terms of blood-clotting from aspirin. And if they did get any benefit it would only be in the area of what we would call platelet aggregation—which is a tiny piece of the blood-clotting story—and not in the coagulation area. So when we get excited about EDTA chelation therapy, what we like is the fact that it works as a synergist with other things in our body.

Most people are vaguely aware that if you have a big blood clot doctors can use Heparin to treat it. Heparin is a natural part of our body's blood-clotting control system and is used to prevent clots. Unfortunately, we normally don't have enough Heparin—the natural anti-clotting, anticoagulant factor present in all human bodies—to handle the acute situation when a heart attack is evolving. This is why people have been trained to rush to the hospital these days to get a Heparin-like treatment known as a tissue plasmogen activator, which can dissolve a clot. But we'd prefer to prevent the clot. For preventing blood clots we have found, miraculously, that if we use a particular form of carrageenan in the presence of EDTA, then synergistically it permits these molecules in our diet to work as a true anti-clotting substance.

Otherwise many people are forced to take a very dangerous drug because they have heart arrhythmias, etc. We selected this form of carrageenan after spending almost ten million dollars researching this. EDTA can actually work synergistically with various food molecules—such as certain kinds of seaweed substances called mucopolysaccharides, like those we would find in red algae called carrageenan—to help prevent blood clots. Carrageenans are mucopolysaccharides—poly meaning "multiple" and "saccharide" meaning "sugar." EDTA and mucopolysaccharides—such as carrageenan from red algae—actually offer dramatic protection from blood clots.

It took over twenty years to get the correct formula, which came out of the ten million dollars worth of research done by Lester Morrison when he was the head of the Institute for Arteriosclerosis Research at La Malinda. Morrison wrote three books on this subject explaining the dramatic benefits. However, in his research he had only looked at it from the viewpoint of a food supplement or a mucopolysaccharide from red algae, and he was having to take a large quantity—like almost a third of a glass of this fiber-like carrageenan material in order to get all of the benefits. When we found that EDTA made this work far more efficiently, we were able to get it down to some convenient capsules. One simply takes three capsules twice a day. And that is actually the history of Essential Daily Defense, a small part of how the oral chelation story came to be.

David: How does EDTA affect nitric oxide levels in the body?

Dr. Gordon: The mechanism by which EDTA affects nitric oxide levels works like this. It has to do with the levels of lead that accumulate in all of our tissues and everyone today is toxic with lead. Clair Patterson from the California Institute of Technology carefully drilled down into the ice cores of the Arctic and Antarctic to find out when we poisoned our nest. In other words, when did we poison the Earth? In order to find that out he had to drill down into the ice, and he found out that human beings are so filthy with lead today that he had to put his researchers in space suits so that they wouldn't contaminate the ice core samples. This is because one drop of sweat, a drop from a nasal secretion, a flake of dead skin, or a piece of hair, is so filled with lead that it wrecks his experiments.

If you look at the Periodic Table of Elements you will see that the atomic structure of lead and zinc are directly related to each other. When you realize how much lead we have in our bodies you begin to see the problem. You see, as we raise the levels of lead we are actually plugging lead into key enzymes functions in our body that normally zinc would have fulfilled. Some of those enzymes are called nitric oxide syntheses. That's multiple because there are several forms of these. Nitric oxide syntheses are the key enzymes that are responsible for this job of attempting to help our body keep a healthy balance of blood flow by making nitric oxide out of the arginine and related amino acids that we get in our diet.

David: Can you talk about EDTA's antiviral and antioxidant activity?

Dr. Gordon: EDTA is a powerful antioxidant that fights free radicals. The Dow chemical company has a huge center on EDTA. They have many different forms of EDTA and they explain a lot in their carefully worded documents. They add EDTA to a number of food products, such as a Chick-fil-A® cole slaw that is widely sold in this country. They buy EDTA by the railroad car because the FDA allows them to make the clear-cut statement that EDTA binds to transition metals, such as copper and iron in any food stuff, as well as these other undesirable metals that we can not avoid.

Every blade of grass and every plant—even those plants growing at a ten thousand foot elevation today—are loaded with lead, mercury, and cadmium from the fallout of the particulate matter from the air that we breathe, which is going directly into our bodies. We find that the radio isotopes from China are actually present in the birds on Mount Washington in America at a ten thousand foot elevation. We can find this in the birds because it's in their diet. It's coating all the foodstuff that everybody eats. So as we begin to realize that all these heavy metals are impossible to avoid, then we can start to see how it became essential to have a way to fight back and the EDTA is the best way that I've been able to find.

EDTA is so safe that you would almost have to drown somebody in it in order to adversely effect them. What's interesting is that Procter & Gamble was looking at topically applied chelators to the skin. They developed one and found that the animals that used it were living twenty percent longer. Now that's important because it suggests that if you're a researcher, and you have an animal eating what you think is a healthy diet, and if you merely chelate that animal by topically applying a chelator to the skin, you can stop free radicals.

Now metals are in everybody. They're everywhere. So what does Dow allow you to say? It says that if you bring EDTA into the equation you tie up these transition metals. Now transition metals are metals that have more than one valiance state. They can be a plus 2 or a plus 3, but all metals catalyze free radicals. So if you really want a powerful antioxidant, then EDTA would truly be the strongest of them all because it has the ability to tie up every metal. If you're a scientist doing research you would have to learn how to get all of the trace elements out of any solution, and even the cleanest water you can buy still has some lead in it until its gone through really rigorous purification measures to be ultra-clean.

Ultra-clean water can cost you hundreds of dollars for a liter of it. So it's kind of interesting that the antioxidant effect of EDTA is directly due to the fact that free metals cause free radicals. EDTA will tie up the metals in solution so that they're no longer free. Remember, I'm using the example of the tablet I give to the dog that I hide in the middle of the hamburger. If you look at it technically, at the atomic level, an atom of lead, copper, or iron is surrounded by the hexidentate, which is the configuration of the EDTA and the way that all of the molecules of EDTA line up. We have really good books with the pictures showing how that works. So the concept of EDTA being an antioxidant is beyond any question.

The antiviral activity, however, is less well documented. But it's important that we get this concept in because, of course, today we're teaching people that heart disease has not so much to do with the cholesterol—like everybody is being told because it sells lots of Lipitor® and lots of other drugs—but much more to do with inflammation. Inflammation is due to many things, but one of the things that clearly it is due to is our low level infections due to the total burden of pathogens. This includes chlamydia, Epstein-Barr, herpes, SB-40, and the list goes on and on. No one today is free of these infections. The book *Plague Time* by Paul Ewald—a professor of theoretical medicine at Amherst and a frequent consultant to PBS—documents the fact that doctors do not even diagnose the chlamydia in everybody today because you can't cure it.

If I give you an antibiotic, you lower the pathogen levels. But when I stop giving you the antibiotic, it comes back because we are all living under unhealthy conditions. So our body is unable to remain free of pathogens. You could take an antibiotic, but of course it will have side-effects. If they keep you on an antibiotic for nine months you will lower some of the body's total burden of bacteria pathogens, but, of course, everybody knows viruses are smarter than bacteria. Now antiviral activity is a low-level property of EDTA and it is not the first substance you think of when you want to lower somebody's burden of herpes, Epstein-Barr, or some of what we call retro-viruses in every person adequately tested today. But it costs around $5000 to give even a semblance of adequate testing to determine pathogen levels in people that want to be tested for all these infections. It costs a fortune to monitor a person's body to find out which ones are present and at what level of activity, but antiviral and antioxidant actions are some of the dramatic benefits EDTA offers.

David: Can you talk about the difference between calcium EDTA and other forms of EDTA?

Dr. Gordon: Yes. With all of the research out there, there will be people that will be more interested in the sodium EDTA. We emphasized the use of sodium EDTA when I wrote the first book with Morton Walker called *The Chelation Answer* because, as an expert in aging, I've been very sensitive to the fact that we appear to be killed by calcium. That sounds like a strong statement with people being told to take calcium, but those of us who are in the know will tell you, without question, the way to kill any nerve cell is to put it in a solution of glutamate and calcium.

Glutamate is a very important part of things that go on in our body, and one is unable to entirely avoid glutamate because it is a part of our diet. Doctors even prescribe it because it helps heal the stomach. Foods from parmesan cheese to tomatoes and peas all wind up producing glutamate in your body. Unfortunately, the glutamate is what we say sets the gun, and when you add calcium it pulls the trigger. It takes the two of them—the glutamate and calcium—to kill nerve cells. Everybody kind of understands that the older they get the weaker their bones are and they become more and more demineralized—yet any doctor doing radiology will tell you that the older the person is the easier it is to see the calcium accumulation on the person's blood vessels. In some people you can see the blood vessels even without putting dye inside the body because there's so much calcium lining our arteries.

What is average? At age eighty you will have on your aorta—the main blood vessel coming out of your heart—one hundred forty times more calcium that it had at age ten. So, in a sense, it almost becomes like a piece a PVC pipe. When you do an autopsy you actually have to have shears to remove the heart from the dead person because the aorta is such a rigid pipe that you need the shears to cut through it. I have spent my life teaching what things like boron, exercise, magnesium, and adequate levels of vitamin K-2 and vitamin D do—that's all covered on my Web site under the word "calcification" or "calcinosis" or "pathologic calcification." So, it would sound then as though nobody would ever want to use calcium EDTA if calcium is such a bad guy.

But we get to some other issues here. We use the sodium EDTA because if you look at the ascending order for which particular atoms EDTA likes—which is well-proven in analytical chemistry—you see that there are certain ones that it likes more than others. EDTA is a weak chelater for things like calcium and magnesium, and it is a powerful chelator for things like lead, mercury, cadmium, and chromium. By weak or strong we mean how strong or weak is the affinity between the EDTA and these various substances. We used sodium EDTA, and we put it in people's veins because we knew that it loved calcium enough that it would make calcium in your body relatively scarce during the time we gave you a sodium chelation I.V. treatment. In other words, if I bubbled it into your arm through an I.V. tube, giving it a drip over a four hour period, during that time the calcium in your blood stream would go down to half normal levels—which would scare some doctors. They would say, my goodness, your going to kill this patient if you don't have any calcium.

You do need calcium in the blood in order to enable a muscle to contract, so obviously by lowering it that much the body says wow, this is pretty hard and pretty scary. The body then reacts by tripling the output of a gland called the parathyroid, which puts out a little parathormone. This then causes the body to put calcium back into solution, making it available to then replace the calcium that I have temporarily tied up with the EDTA.

So this means that the EDTA has temporarily got a new partner, and they're dancing through the blood vessels. However, this is not a partner that the EDTA wants to have for life, because EDTA really would prefer lead for a lifetime partner. Other metals, like zinc, it just likes a lot. So, because people have these hard rigid arteries that are lined with calcium, what we realized is that if we could put some of that calcium back into the solution then sodium EDTA was a good choice. However, sodium EDTA did not go in the arm painlessly. It actually causes some aching, some pain, and a little spasm of the vessels, so it can sometimes be difficult to sit in a chair for four hours.

Now, that would be okay if you could really have everyone reliably do that. Every person will have a huge benefit. If you could make all the plaque on people's arteries go away then they won't ever need bypass surgery. But they need to be sitting in the chair for four hours thirty times, fifty times, or a hundred times. Many patients have needed a hundred chelations. I.V. Chelation therapy is very safe. In the over ten million people treated with intravenous chelation there haven't been any deaths. So it wasn't a bad deal, but you have to measure that against the following facts. We did see an improvement in blood flow in eighty-six percent of the patients treated. They could walk farther, go up hills or more flights of stairs, have less leg cramps and chest pain, better vision, and lots of dramatic things happened.

We treated ten million people. After enough time went by we became aware that although we had improved blood flow, we hadn't really gotten all the junk out of the artery. So then we had to sit back and say, wait a minute. The person is getting a dramatic benefit. He thinks I'm a genius. But in some cases we actually witnessed that the blockage in the artery had increased. In some cases it had been at sixty percent when we started treatment and was now up to a seventy percent blockage. You sit there and say, wait a minute, how can that be? My arteries are actually more blocked but I'm now able to jog again. I can play golf again. I can run up stairs again. What's going on?

Obviously it gets really complicated inside the human body. A lot of the blood vessels are what we call collateral, and they are very tiny, like capillaries. They can not be seen on an arteriogram. So what really happens in the body needs sophisticated testing, not the outdated arteriogram on people that have been cut open. Every year we cut open half a million people doing some kind of surgery based on a totally misleading test called an angiogram, which only looks at the highway and doesn't look at the detour sites around a blocked artery. A detour site would be like if you went through the farmer's field. It's a dirt road, but it gets around the obstruction and everybody gets to St. Louis on time. Then you didn't need to have such a big fuss about the obstruction. So in order to find that you need a PET scan.

A PET scan is expensive, and its not widely available, so people continue to be operated on for nonurgent reasons, because what they can see on the arteries is never actually what's going to kill you. In fact, it's so sad. The plaque that kills you doesn't show up in the angiogram because it's in the wall of the vessel. But that's another topic. That's under the topic "vulnerable plaque." The patients that were getting the sodium EDTA could lower the pathologic calcium in their blood vessels but we didn't get rid of all the plaque. So then we had to sit there and say, what is going on?

Finally, after thirty years of banging our heads against the wall, we began to realize that lead has more of a toxic effect on the body than we had ever dreamed. When we started we knew that any form of chelation—calcium EDTA, sodium EDTA, magnesium EDTA, all of these—would grab lead, but, at the time, we never really believed that lead, mercury, and cadmium were such a big problem for human beings. So we ignored the obvious. Then we finally realized, hey wait a minute, if we use the calcium EDTA then it's entirely painless. We can give the treatment in three or four minutes and you're out of the office and back to work. So it doesn't cost you four hours of your productive income, and you're not paying the doctor a huge sum of money to have to be observed by competent people while an I.V. is running in your arm.

So it was win-win. What happened was we became aware that because the EDTA was painlessly administered, we could get it in fast enough to get it up to a higher level of concentration. The sodium EDTA was so painful that you had to administer it very slow—drip, drip, drip—so the calcium EDTA going in rapidly was actually more like a deep wax Simonize® than a wash job. If you administered the sodium EDTA you were helping everybody, but weren't getting a deep cleansing of the lead, mercury, and cadmium.

Then we began to wake up to the fact that clearing the body of the heavy metals themselves was the primary reason that people could now run up the stairs, because of nitric oxide and things related to that. Also, EDTA improves blood viscosity, or the thickness of the blood, which I haven't mentioned yet. If your blood is thick like honey you can't walk up and down steps. If it's thin like wine you can walk up and down just fine. But those are all different topics. All these different forms of EDTA confuse people. I have finally gotten people to wake up to the fact that calcium EDTA works at least as well as the sodium EDTA. That was a shock because ten million people sat in the chair as I did for four hours, taking up a lot of valuable time with an aching arm. Now, worldwide, more and more doctors are switching to calcium EDTA. Calcium EDTA, by the way, is added by the ton to our food, but it's only added in enough quantities to protect the food from spoiling.

Now I've raised the level so that we take it in supplements and get enough—not only to protect the garlic and the other things that are in the supplements from ever turning bad—but also enough to protect the human body. So just like Dow® is legally allowed to tell people that they add their EDTA to foodstuff to prevent spoiling, I tell every one of my patients that I don't want them to spoil on me either. Everybody knows that we have all kinds of substances that have been used in an effort to prevent spoilage, but most people never think about their body spoiling. There is this process called lipid peroxidation—when fats turn rancid—and everybody may have heard by now that if fat is rancid it can kill your dog if you give it to him. So you don't keep things around that are rancid.

What I'm trying to teach people is that EDTA does many things, and we have to have enough in our body at all times. Just think of the intestinal tract itself. There is more bacteria in your intestine than there are cells in your body. There are a lot of biochemical reactions going on and technically some of those bacteria are responsible for converting your food into useful nutrients. For example, B-6, folic acid, and some vitamin K are not in their active form until they're acted upon in the gut. But if you don't tie up and protect the human body from interactions with the toxic metals that are in our water, food, and air, then you have a lot of free radicals going on in your intestines. This is why we have a needless epidemic of colon cancer.

My position is very simple. Many people attack the use of oral chelation that utilizes any form of EDTA. They say that when you put EDTA in your veins it is a hundred percent absorbed and I can't deny that. It clearly is, and in one four hour infusion you can get some of the same benefits you might get from a month of using the oral form of EDTA. But even if you never wanted to take the oral form of EDTA, you would be well-advised to take some every day because of the epidemic of colon cancer today—because it is the interaction between various molecules in your intestinal tract that wind up with what we call oxidized biosalts that can lead to the formation of very toxic substances.

These very toxic substances wind up inside ninety-nine percent of all people in America today. When we test people's bowel movements we find carcinogens and mutagens in their feces. These people are bathing their poor colon in substances that are so toxic that it's wonder that everybody doesn't get colon cancer. By merely adding EDTA you prevent all of those lipid peroxidases and other reactions from going on because you are eliminating the metals that catalyze those bad reactions.

So I have my bias with calcium EDTA because its well tolerated. I've already said these nasty things about calcium, and how much I don't like taking tons of calcium supplements every day because its not the answer that everybody's being told. If you look at Chinese peasants they have strong bones at age ninety and they have a total daily intake of calcium at approximately a third of what we get in our diet. So people are not in need of calcium, but they're being lied to for complex reasons, and it's a great business. But what we want to have is the idea that the calcium EDTA that I've chosen to use in both the I.V. and oral is there for a specific purpose to do a specific job. In the form of the I.V. it's because it's painless, allowing me to get a high enough concentration to really do a deep cleansing and move a lot of lead out of the person's body in a short time. This makes it more economical and cost effective.

In the oral form, amazingly enough I'm still getting a win-win because, like it or not, every human being in America does have to take some calcium supplementation, even though I don't like it, because we have so much phosphorus in our diet—from soft drinks and the high ingestion of meat. So when you look at my work on pathologic calcification as a cause of aging you will see that I tell people that they don't need that much calcium. When you look at the health-assessment nutrition evaluation by the United States government and the NIH, and if you read all their papers, you'll see that the average person gets 1300 milligrams of phosphorus and about 800 milligrams of calcium per day.

So I have to give you about four or five hundred milligrams of calcium a day. So in my oral form of chelation you're only getting roughly sixty, seventy, eighty milligrams of calcium, so it's not going to perturb the balance in the wrong way. I'm bringing in the EDTA that I do need in a form that is able to move lead out of people's bodies. And the amount of lead that comes out has been researched by Los Alamos Research Laboratory, and even they scratch their head, and say, wait a minute, how does this work out?

Let's talk about I.V. for the moment, because it's a hundred percent absorbed. Oral EDTA is only five to eighteen percent absorbed, but in fact it was the oral that actually got Los Alamos concerned. They said look, if this stuff is only five to eighteen percent absorbed how come the children that we give it to have so much lead coming out of their body?

A lot of people laugh at you and think you're stupid for using calcium

EDTA orally. Don't you know that it's only five to eighteen percent absorbed? What we're suggesting is that by having the non-absorbed calcium EDTA, maybe not only am I protecting myself against colon cancer, but maybe by having it in my intestines at all times it's acting almost as a magnet, a sponge, or an ionic exchange resin, causing some of the lead, mercury, and cadmium that is in my blood at all times. Remember my blood is washing through all those little tiny blood vessels, bathing my intestinal tract in that side of the thin vessel, the capillary. There is the bad lead and inside of my intestine there's that nice high safe concentration of EDTA.

When we do fecal analysis of heavy metals on our autistic children, we find out that in fact feces may be one of the major ways that we're getting heavy metals out of people, although, of course, we have all the children and all the adults who are willing to, also bathe regularly in EDTA, because the skin is another route of excretion. If you sat in a sauna and you collected your sweat, you would see that your sweat is another major route of getting the mercury and lead out.

So that's a long answer to a simple question. But the forms of EDTA that are out there each have their own place, and there is nothing wrong with somebody being an advocate of something like magnesium EDTA. But the problem is that it's not widely available commercially, and I do not trust the sources of supply. So the companies that have chosen to sell magnesium EDTA I do not get involved with because they are not on the safe ground as they would be with the calcium EDTA. Using calcium EDTA with Lester Morrison's formula of the mucopolysaccharide allows people to go twenty years without a fatal heart attack. I'm so confident today that I cancel bypass surgery on anybody who calls me.

I don't care if they're eighty to ninety percent obstructed, or if they're a world famous television personality. I simply say, well, if your time comes then your time has come, but it's been twenty years and so far we don't ever see anybody dropping dead of a heart attack who's using the total program that I call oral chelation. This involves omega-3 fatty acids, garlic, primrose, and lots of things beyond EDTA—but in a symphony. I would never administer this program to anybody without EDTA being a key part of the symphony.

David: Why is EDTA suspected to stimulate mitochondrial activity?

Dr. Gordon: I've cogitated that for a long time. It was my eighth chelation treatment when, for the first time in my life, I was able to run up a two thousand foot elevation. That would be approximately three and half miles up a steep road, and I didn't even start to tire at the top of it, while a two year old Irish Setter had it's tongue hanging down to the ground. The chelation treatments turned me into Superman. So how could that happen after just the eighth treatment?

In those days—thirty-four or thirty-five years ago—I was dumb enough to think that maybe I'd found the cardiovascular equivalent of Drano® and that the chelation treatments were dissolving arterial blockages. I knew that by the age of twenty-one all of the young men killed in Korea and Vietnam always had lots of arteriosclerosis. So I just assumed that because I'd had disabling angina by the age of twenty-nine that maybe I had found a Roto-Rooter® that cleaned all my vessels. I didn't really think about the mitochondria at that time. Then I started working with a company called Wakunaga in Japan, and they had a form of oral chelation using some garlic substances. We started to look at mitochondrial function because they wound up giving large doses of this oral chelation formula to their handball team, and they became the top handball team in Japan.

It became clear that there was a tremendous increase in energy. Then when you start talking to people who do nothing but study mitochondrial function, they'll tell you that heavy metals tend to congregate at the outer membrane level of the mitochondria and they're significantly impeding the ability for you to make the currency of energy which is called ATP (adenosine triphosphate). So if we begin to study that function it becomes very clear that any time you can remove that lead you'll experience dramatic benefits and you don't have to get it all out of your body. This is the most incredible thing about this whole conversation.

Let's look at the work by Harid Hardy at Mass. General, published in one of the journals of occupational medicine twenty-five or thirty years ago. She was astonished by the recovery of a patient who had come to see her. He had been a painter and he had what we call "Alner Nerve Dropping." This means that a nerve had died in his arm and part of his arm was useless. It had been that way for around five or ten years. She put him on chelation and in less then two months this whole nerve function in his arm came back.

What we've had to learn since then is that it takes fifteen years to remove all of the lead from an adult's bones. It takes children around five to seven years to do this using chelation therapy.

So obviously the chelation she gave the patient could not have started to have removed all the lead, because, after all, you are born with a significant level of lead. This is because, as a rapidly growing tissue inside of a mother's body, the mother's body assumes you are a waste basket. So the mother's body takes the lead and mercury out of her system and dumps it into the baby. This is why six hundred thousand children a year are born with mercury toxicity in the United States, according to the EPA.

So lead poisoning is in everybody. Now, if we look at it then, how in the world can all that mitochondrial function and energy happen? Well, some people have a defect in their enzyme functioning which we call COMT—. If you have a gene for methyl transferase that's negative (-) then you don't get rid of these heavy metals at all. So these people still function but they're all able to function far better with chelation.

Then you have the inner current poisoning that goes on. My father was an orthopedic physician and surgeon and he was lied to by three different dentists. Each one who saw me said that the last guy put in all my mercury fillings wrong. Then they would drill them all out and put in all new mercury fillings. In other words, it was called a sucker game and they just about killed me. After the third dentist I had narcolepsy, hypoglycemia, and I was so sick that I could hardly function. I had acute mercury toxicity from it going way beyond genes into actual things that had been put into my body. And if you look at that it would only make sense then to have a dramatic reversal.

This, by the way, is the toughest part of this oral chelation story. The Dow documents are in my slides from the talk that I gave at Cancer

Control. I strongly recommend that you look at the presentations on my Web site. One is called "Cancer Control" and the other one is "IACN," and that's the International Academy of Clinical Nutrition.

In those two presentations the important slide was when Dow shows exactly how many atoms of mercury or lead can be handled by how much EDTA. It is astonishing and it's a subject of major controversy worldwide. It shows that lead and mercury are the two most effective substances to be tied by EDTA. Now what does "tied up" mean? It means it's bound. Being bound is essentially, for all practical purposes, like being in a shell game. It's out of sight and out of mind, out of harm's way. Even though it hasn't yet taken the lead or mercury out of your body, by tying it up the mercury can no longer interfere with the production of glutathione in your body, among the thousands of things that it does.

So we just need to realize that the ability to get a chelating agent to nullify the toxic effect of these heavy metals is sufficient in and of itself, but it's very confusing to the poor patients, because we have patients who continue to die after seeing an average chelation doctor. We have patients die because doctors really are confused. They say, well, we gave you thirty treatments. When you came here you couldn't walk ten feet and now you're able to jog five miles so we must have helped. We'll see you around. They don't realize that as soon they stop the treatments they have not cured the patient. If the patient took those treatments over the course of a year then the patient has only got rid of one fifteenth of the total lead from his body, which, in the long run, is not a big enough bang to have a long-term benefit—even though he now feels great because you've essentially neutralized the enemy.

But the enemy is hiding, waiting to come out again as soon as they stop the chelating. This is why it's so sad. I have very bright doctors who are helping a lot of people with intravenous chelation that feel fantastically improved—but they don't understand two things. They feel improved but they didn't get the cleaning of their arteries that they had hoped to get.

We've treated ten million people. Because arteriosclerosis is in and of itself a disease that is not always static, and is remodeling itself constantly, you have more at some times and a little less at other times. Out of all those we have some people that look like we dramatically cleaned their arteries but that's not the average story. If we look at the average story we realize that people are getting this increase in energy at the mitochondrial level, so the guy now has the energy to run up and down the steps because he increased his efficiency.

Let's look at what we call the "ejection fraction," that is—how strong can your heart contract? When I have a heart that really squeezes down tight, that's ideal, and sixty, seventy, eighty percent of the blood that's in the heart is ejected. But when it's flabby and you're ready to die then it's down to around a thirty percent ejection, meaning it's hardly pushing any blood out.

We have dramatic pictures of people whose hearts were filling their whole lung cavity. They were living on oxygen machines and we got them all breathing again. We turned many people around, but we have to be careful to realize, that just because we turned them around doesn't mean that we cleared their arteries.

In his book *The Sinatra Solution*, Steve Sinatra—who doesn't even use chelation—says that he's routinely canceling heart transplants. I have been able to cancel every heart transplant, because I use all the things that Steve talks about—the carnitine, the alpha lipoic acid, and the ribose—in addition to chelation. The ribose, the magnesium, and the coenzyme Q-10 are important. Ribose is a big story. It is a five carbon sugar. Normally we're against sugar, but here's a sugar that takes no effort for the body to convert into the currency of energy called ATP.

So that's another arrow in our quiver which allows us to treat sicker and sicker people faster and faster by adding these additional things I just rattled off for the treatment of heart disease. It's important to realize that mitochondrial function is critical. In addition to EDTA there are many things—from carnitine to coenzyme Q-10—that are going to enhance mitochondrial function. But clearly it helps if you can get some of the heavy metals tied up so they're no longer effectively preventing ATP production. Again, when we think of it, always think of the simplest example. Lead competes in the body with zinc and zinc is a catalyst to many enzymes. Whenever you have an enzyme that is not operating efficiently you have a less than efficient production of biochemical reactions and the person is not operating optimally.

David: I'm curious about how chelation therapy effects the brain. How has EDTA been shown to help improve memory, enhance concentration and act as an antidepressant?

Dr. Gordon: Let's start by looking at the work on people who have been poisoned by heavy metals and all the literature on lead workers. The highest rate of suicide was among dentists. This was because dentists all worked with mercury. They were never warned about the danger of mercury. Lead poisoning was also called Mad Hatter Syndrome. This is because lead, mercury, and cadmium all have unique areas in the brain that they target and they knock out certain neurotransmitters. The production of dopamine, serotonin and all the other feel-good neurotransmitters are entirely dependent on efficient enzymatic activity. So any person that you take the lead out of today gives them energy and improves the biochemical mixture in their brain.

I've been involved in studying trace metals now for thirty-five years and our research reveals that we can always find aluminum, cadmium, mercury, and lead in the plaque that is part of Alzheimer's disease, multiple sclerosis, etc. So as we start to put all these pieces together we see that all of these toxins have an effect on biochemical levels and that is always going to have a psychiatric equivalent, as well as an energy equivalent. In this discussion I've focused on the energy equivalent— because, obviously, if your heart is beating strong and you can climb up steps, that is a useful thing. But your brain has also got to process information efficiently, and it is not doing that when the enzymes that are critical in the brain for neurotransmitters like dopamine, serotonin, and noradrenaline are knocked out and not operating efficiently.

David: Why doesn't EDTA remove important metals and minerals from the body, such as zinc, and why is it essential to take a multi mineral while on an EDTA program?

Dr. Gordon: EDTA is not smart enough to be able to go in the body and say, oh I'm just going to take you out and I don't take you out. So EDTA will cause as much as a hundredfold increase in the excretion of zinc.

As doctors we have felt that it's certainly necessary to replace that zinc, especially because so many people obtain only a marginal intake of zinc from their diet to begin with.

There's a nice textbook picture in Dr. Bruce Alstead's book that shows EDTA's mechanisms of action and I've written about it extensively. So, yes, EDTA has always got the theoretical risk that you could become copper deficient, and if you use a lot of DMSA you can clearly become zinc deficient. But what's confusing about this is the following. The body has a lot of innate wisdom, so if your body becomes mineral or metal deficient, it seems that it is able to ramp up the efficiency with which it absorbs minerals like calcium and metals like zinc.

Some of the early doctors didn't give their patients mineral supplements with chelation. Dr. Norman Clarke at Providence Hospital in Detroit, Michigan, was really the first doctor to ever actually get involved in EDTA research and he published the first study on it, although he never bothered to give zinc to anybody. When he was ninety-one years of age he bounced up on the lectern to address all the doctors when I invited him to speak. I had been kind of embarrassed because he was ninety-one and I thought that I was going to help this old guy get up on the thing because it was about a three foot jump, but he just jumped up there. So obviously he'd been taking his own chelation. And I was this young guy trying to convince him that I knew more about EDTA than him and he needs to be taking zinc. He never took zinc and he wouldn't take a multiple.

He took the attitude that we get rid of a lot of old zinc and the body then is wise enough to bring in new zinc if you're eating intelligently. But since the literature would make a doctor taking that attitude at great risk, and because of our own research with rat pups, we chose to always supplement with zinc and other minerals during chelation. Our studies showed that when we gave EDTA to a rat mother we could get malformations in the rat pups unless we gave zinc. So I have always advocated that we must replace zinc. But that's not a very hard thing to do. I have been on oral chelation for over thirty years, and I have many patients who have been on it for over twenty-five years. Frankly, it is a very simple thing. In a sense, it's almost like the old metals may have given up some of their electrons, or their usefulness, and the body is happy to see the new metals come in.

There was a time when people only went out and bought vitamins instead of vitamins with minerals. And there was a time that companies like Theragran-M® with Squibb® cheated the public and sold them a product as magnesium supplements that on the label said epsom salts. Once you discover that epsom salts are actually magnesium sulfate you realize that it actually robs the body of magnesium. So it's nice if you pay attention and get a really good product that somebody has paid attention to, and just because something says on the label it has zinc, copper, or magnesium in it doesn't mean they care about whether it really works in your body.

David: If EDTA is removing calcium, then how does it affect bone growth?

Dr. Gordon: The interesting thing is that when you take the disodium EDTA it actually stimulates bone growth. Disodium EDTA is the intravenous compound that I initially championed. What happens to people as they age is that their blood vessels turn to stone. Let's give it a number. At age ten you have a certain amount of calcium in your aorta. At age eighty there will be a hundred forty times more calcium in every person's aorta.

So with disodium EDTA, you actually tie up the calcium that's in the blood, so that the body thinks there's a shortage of calcium, and it turns on the parathyroid hormone. The parathyroid hormone then mobilizes that calcium that has been building up in your artery. Provably, we can lower that content of calcium in your vascular tissue, and, amazingly enough, that same parathyroid hormone switch will make you turn on bone growth again. It's a very exciting process. After all, we're the only medical society with two practicing ninety-four year old members. They've had over two thousand intravenous treatments. They have perfectly healthy bones, nice soft arteries, and they are still practicing. They are still able to show up and enjoy working. Anti-aging is part of the chelation treatment. So there's a big difference.

So, because few people could understand everything I just said, we have largely now switched to the calcium EDTA. Calcium EDTA gives you calcium when we give you the EDTA, and it makes it a painless treatment, taking three to five minutes. This cuts down the cost of the treatment from $120 to around $60, making it available to everybody, because it doesn't interfere with their day's productivity. People can swing by the doctor's office, be in there five minutes, and have the treatment. The treatment is given rapidly, because it's painless, and it will take out as much as ten or twenty times more lead per treatment than we get out of the old treatment. But it doesn't do that interesting thing that I've talked about of lowering the level of calcium in your arteries, and enhancing the uptake of calcium in your bone, which is done under the parathyroid hormone influence. In fact, if you are a world expert on parathyroid hormone, you'll know that disodium EDTA infusions are called parathyroid tropic hormones.

The old treatment, that we've treated ten million people safely with— without a known death—is the treatment used in the Trial to Access Chelation Therapy (TACT) study done by the National Institutes of Health. The TACT study, funded for twenty-nine million dollars, is studying the old treatment that I brought to the world. Ten million people have had the benefits of that therapy, and about eighty-five percent of them said they saw enough improvement in their circulation that allowed them to avoid a proposed amputation of an extremity, a placement in a nursing home because of loss of vision or memory, or the proposed bypass that some hospital was telling them they needed.

We do not do bypass surgeries. I've done no bypasses on any patient in twenty years. I don't do stents. I cancel all of that surgery based on a simple rule. I ask patients the following question: What are the benefits of the proposed surgery that the hospital or the doctor wants to do, and what are the risks? Once people understand that the benefit is extremely weak, and the risks are extremely large, then they can choose to bet their life on what I'm telling them. There has not yet been a single known fatality in twenty years among people who are simply taking EDTA, and I canceled surgery on people who have eighty to ninety percent blocked vessels.

David: What are some other effective chelators besides EDTA?

Dr. Gordon: The world is filled with chelators. Tetracycline, vitamin C, and lactic acid are chelators. Exercise is a chelator.

David: Tetracycline? Do you mean the antibiotic?

Dr. Gordon: Yes, it sure is. See, that's what is so confusing for a lot of people. We have lots of people who categorize a drug in a particular way and people think that's all it does. Let's say you're talking about Dilantin®, which is used by many people to control epilepsy. Well, what if it stops a totally different condition, like when you're fearful of heights, agoraphobia. Then, obviously, you need to understand that it might be a basement membrane stabilizer. So what I'm trying to drive at here is that we have some very confusing information going on because a drug that is listed as an anti-yeast drug may also be a chelator. So we have people really confused in this medical world. Some people assume that if a drug they took was helpful in controlling seizures, and you got better, then you must have had some kind of an undiagnosed seizure disorder. So always it turns out that everything works on many levels and antibiotics are chelators.

But let's try to remember that it would take fifteen years of consistent, without fail, chelating to remove all the toxic heavy metals from someone's body. One needs to be pushing the lead, mercury, copper, and cadmium out of their body—excreting it through the feces, the sweat, and the urine—for fifteen years. So it doesn't make a lot of difference in a sense, but I don't want people to assume that tetracycline would be the great answer. It's important to understand that one of the ways that many antibiotics work is through chelation.

So let's go to the top of the page again. Apple acid, malic acid, great chelators. Garlic, great chelator. In fact, these are the ones that I use. I make a joke of it and tell everybody that I'm just your friendly truck farmer. I have everybody taking my better grown EDTA. I have everybody on apple acid, because malic acid is needed for everything that we do. And I have everybody on garlic. So you begin to get the idea that I really believe these are great foods.

Garlic is such a great chelator. But when the head of a company in Japan wanted to find a place to grow garlic I had to admit to him that any garlic that you raise in the central valley of California—if it's within a quarter of the mile of the freeway—is going to be contaminated with lead because all freeways throw trash into the surrounding dirt.

In New Zealand it is so dangerous to have your cow eat the grass that's next to the road because your cow is going to get lead poisoning. This is because New Zealand doesn't have the newer methods of refineries that we have that are relatively low lead. They have high-lead refineries, and all the gas is loaded with lead. So any car going down the street is passing cadmium out from the wearing of tires and lead from the exhaust. So if you're a chelator it's really nice to have people test what they sell you. Every product that we are involved in we measure the level of lead, arsenic, mercury, etc., because so much of our agriculture is contaminated. A single cabbage that is grown just a hundred yards from a freeway in California can contain a thousand times the safe level of cadmium as a result of being next to a freeway.

David: Can you talk about some of the most recent studies that have been done with EDTA?

Dr. Gordon: The big study that's going on now is the Trial to Access Chelation Therapy—otherwise known as the TACT study—and it's supposed to be funded to the tune of twenty-nine million dollars. Currently, it's less than halfway through its five year study. The study is merely to test one thing—will people who use some chelation with an oral vitamin and mineral supplement during those five years have less heart attacks, or less of need for surgery, than the people who got a placebo? That was the question that the Trial to Access Chelation Therapy put up.

This study is not near and dear to me because it's using the old outdated sodium EDTA that requires four hour treatments, which nobody really has time for anymore, and the study really came out of my incorrect belief thirty years ago that I found Nirvana. I thought I had found the magic bullet to clean everybody's arteries and we now know that we don't have it. So since I'm really much more focused on the long-term implications today, I'm sorry to see us waste our money on a study that only does a few chelations and then follows subjects for a few years.

It will probably come out as a slight benefit, but nowhere near the kind of benefit that one is able to achieve if people are put on to the oral chelation after the I.V.s. I have nothing against I.V. I love I.V. chelation. It's always going to be good. Asking if I was against I.V. chelation would be like asking, would I be against Simonizing my car. I'm never against a deep cleansing, but the problem is I need to wash the car every day for the next fifty years in addition to the Simonizing. So that's the problem.

We've got the Simonizing and the washing confused. So we have some people saying, oh I took the I.V.s and that's all I need. Well, that's not all they need, and they still can drop dead on you.

David: Why isn't oral EDTA chelation recommended by more physicians?

Dr. Gordon: I think this is because the standard policy of doctors is to be down on what they're not up on. You see, the scientific literature in this country is entirely controlled. The net result is that if you have a real breakthrough, something that's really going to cure cancer or heart disease, it's not going to be in the *New England Journal of Medicine* or *Lancet* because of the game that is played in this world. We've known from the beginning that this was too big a revolution. If every doctor did what I'm promoting, there would be no huge hospitals, with huge mills. Every year about four to five hundred thousand people have bypass surgery. That's a huge part of our budget. There's a lot of people dependent on that income, so it's hard to make a big change suddenly, because of the economic ramifications. These changes don't happen suddenly. They happen when people start asking questions. But we've treated ten million people. Those people know, and they've told their families that this actually made them able to go back and run their business, or that this got them out of the nursing home. We have documented so many success stories that it's incredible.

APPENDIX B

AN INTERVIEW WITH LESLIE HAMUD, CNT

BY DAVID JAY BROWN

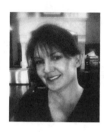 *Leslie Hamud is a certified nutritional therapist (CNT). She is also the mother of two children who suffer from autism, both of whom experienced a significant decrease in symptoms after using detoxification therapy. Leslie and her children live in California. I spoke with Leslie on May 20, 2007. In the excerpt from our conversation below, Leslie talks about the benefits that her children experienced from detoxification therapy.*

David: Can you tell me a little bit about your two children who suffer from autism?

Leslie: I have two boys, thirteen and nine. I was just recalling how, in the beginning, the top neurologist in the state of California, said regarding the oldest, that he would probably grow out of it. I was offered medication if it became too difficult for me to handle. About the third appointment he said, "You know the younger one is higher functioning than the older one." At that point I decided that the medical profession did not know how to handle these children.

You have to remember this was during the years 1999-2001. No one was willing to admit there was indeed a problem. We opted not to choose the course of medications as I did not feel there was enough research with the pharmaceutical agents to justify their use in young children. I also firmly believed that their bodies were still developing. I didn't want to interrupt any more growth or processing than had already been done. With that I decided to take this on myself and started researching.

David: What are the symptoms that they experienced?

Leslie: In the very beginning, we realized there were issues when they both exhibited a speech-delay, visual disruption and separation anxiety. There were sensory integration issues; one of them couldn't tolerate being touched and the other one couldn't sense touch. They were on different ends of the sensory spectrum. My theory was their development was being delayed because the body was dealing with the sludge or toxins on board.

They were both definitely late in talking, and were hard to understand. There was a lot of grunting and pointing as a form of communication. Language was not understood until the ages of six or seven. They were latent in their potty-training and as a result there were some social issues. Sensory integration seemed to be the core of the outburst. Anything having to do with senses was difficult—whether they're eating food, digesting it, the way their clothing feels on their body, the light from the sun and sounds, or differing from hot to cold. Being able to understand and interpret their own nervous system, then responding to it in an appropriate manner, was difficult. There were just a lot of sensory integration issues.

David: Detoxification therapy aside, what are some of the different treatments that you've tried?

Leslie: We first tried standard occupational therapy and speech therapy. Which was very good. It helps if you can work with a person who is a sensory-trained therapist. They are a little more in tune to the complexities of the nervous system. Speech is interesting in that with all the years we did therapy it never took hold. Although once I got them into piano—in particular the grand piano—their speech started to evolve. I feel the vibrations from the piano strings stimulated the language centers of the brain.

David: That's very interesting.

Leslie: Yes, it is. Actually, if you do some research you will find that vibration was our first mode of communication. So, for them, it was about the nervous system being stimulated, and/or not stimulated enough. For one child it was over-stimulation and for the other it was under-stimulation. It was definitely a seesaw effect that I needed to continue to work with. There's no doubt that it helped them. Movement and exploring other sensory experiences is the best thing. In other words, let's get back to recess and encourage them to move!

David: What type of detoxification therapy have you been using?

Leslie: Both of the boys' detox pathways were blocked in the beginning. The only form of therapy that could first be used was sweating, because the methylation pathways were blocked. The first line of defense for the children was the infrared sauna, which I didn't discover for awhile. You have to understand that not much was available on autism in the beginning. There just wasn't anyone giving you any type of informed instruction on detoxing a body. Dr. Garry Gordon, and Dr. Sherri Rogers (the toxicologist from New York), were the only ones who had procedures.

The second step was to include the work of Dr. Amy Yasko. She helped me to understand the importance of methylation pathways and their roles in the body. Once I supported the methylation pathways, then other avenues could participate in the detoxification process. After all, it is what the body is designed to do naturally.

The third approach was simply changing the food supply. When you eliminate toxins from your food and start ingesting pure foods (which are not laden with pesticides and are grown organically with proper attention) all of a sudden the body can do more, and it will start detoxifying on its own. Organic and biodynamically grown foods are the best. Just by doing these two simple things enabled the body to do some form of detoxification, and—again—when you support the methylation pathways then all of a sudden you're accomplishing more.

David: Have you used EDTA chelation therapy?

Leslie: In the beginning they could not do this form of chelation therapy. As the body removed some of the sludge of toxins it freed itself up and there was more room. I started eliminating toxins from their food supply and they became a little more particular about the food they were ingesting. Spending some time in the infrared sauna, you start freeing up the body. All of a sudden the EDTA that once gave you a problem now becomes a resource for the body. They are now able to do two forms of EDTA chelation. One is the EDTA chewing gum and the other is the EDTA bath formula, Beyond Clean.

David: So they're still not orally ingesting it?

Leslie: Well, they do the EDTA gum.

David: But that doesn't really get much of it into their digestive system.

Leslie: This is what you have to also consider. I think that a big component of chelation therapy is first determining if the digestive system is able to take in the nutrients and respond to treatment. For the boys it couldn't. By chewing the gum in the mouth it can enter the body sublingually and/or by soaking the body in the tub it enters the body through the skin, transdermally.

As a CNT, we use an approach called Lingual-Neuro Testing, where the client keeps a vitamin supplement in the mouth and the brain responds to it very quickly. The beauty is in that it is bypassing the stomach. Items like Dr. Gordon's soap, or an EDTA-based gum and some creams are a better option. Especially if a person's digestive tract is so disrupted, and perhaps leaky, that nothing is getting through anyway. It's like you've got this beautiful car (the human body), that's got wonderful alignment (nutritional support), but you're traveling down a bumpy road that has no pavement (the digestive system). Something will give and it will probably be your health.

David: So the primary things that really helped in the very beginning were the infrared sauna and changing the diet. What kind of an effect did those things have?

Leslie: With the infrared sauna, the only thing that I noticed from that was that the boys would come out of the sauna smelling like tin foil.

David: That's interesting that you could actually smell the aluminum leaving their bodies.

Leslie: Then, when I changed their diet, all of a sudden, they became less 'spacey.' As the MSG and other excitotoxins in their food were diminished, that 'spaciness' improved. They developed a better ability to focus, to listen to your words, and take directions. And, gradually, as we continued to support the body and methylation pathways, all the way down the line things improved. 'Down the line' or 'up the ladder', as an occupational therapist would say.

You've got to first have a foundation before you can start building all the skills of walking, talking, running, and jumping. You've got to have a foundation. For me, the infrared sauna, methylation support, EDTA chewing gum, Beyond Clean and nutritional support all help. It's important to remember that each person's 'toxic load' is different. Some people really express their toxic load in their skin, so they may have eczema or certain kinds of skin disorders, but with others it may be expressed neurologically. So you've got to find out each person's individual needs, and what pathway works. Then, once you discover that—run with it. If you continue to work with the pathway that is available then something else will eventually pull into line and open up.

David: How are your children doing now?

Leslie: Honestly, I think they're doing really well. I'd like to see a little more weight on my youngest son. There's still some kidney issues with him and that gives us problems. Whereas the oldest is now five foot six inches and he weighs a hundred fifty pounds. He's got weight on him and of course you know we store toxins in our fat tissue as well. This weight allows his body to have another place to store toxins. This is not to say that he's toxin-free. I mean, every breath we take is full of toxins.

Dr. Gordon put it the best when he said you could spend twenty or thirty thousand dollars to have every test in the world done, which should help you to figure where you're at—but you haven't done a thing to start removing all those toxins from your body. It's better to take that money and just start chipping away at the iceberg. As long as the body is supported via the methylation pathway, and the elimination pathway is open, then products such as EDTA can start to have a positive effect on the body. This is important because when you mobilize toxins you best make sure they're leaving. If toxins are not able to leave the body then it will start manifesting toxins as a disease. Some call it cancer, we called it autism. The digestive tract becomes very important in maintaining health.

So for us, absorbing through the skin was an option, chewing the EDTA gum, and letting all that EDTA sit in the mouth was a big thing and it did help. Then supporting the methylation pathway which is like opening up a freeway really turned things on. I would say in the long run it is all part of the puzzle. If we all address detoxification our minds become sharper, our skin will be more vibrant, our hair will be shinier.

One thing I've noticed with chelation is that the boy's hair texture has definitely changed. Eyes have become clearer and more bright. The skin has become peach-toned, and just more vibrant. The body's gone from this distilled state of toxicity to this vibrant state of health.

It's a process. I don't know that we'll ever be done with it, but it definitely has freed them up neurologically, and that's nice to see. Language did pop in and social abilities did start forming. They developed the ability to know where their limbs are spatially. In your nervous system that's called "mapping," when you can tell where your knee is at without really looking at it. That's the anatomic nervous system bringing back the messaging.

Any time you chelate you're going to free up intercellular and organ activities, and those activities are the basis of life. So when you free them up, the cells can now start dumping the toxins that are inside them, relaying messages and doing all the other cellular activities. Organs—like the liver being the primary king—can start doing their job, such as breaking down carbohydrates, fats, and proteins. The liver helps to maintain a normal blood sugar level. It also stores some vitamins and, in particular, activates vitamin D. The kidneys can start doing their job excreting wastes through the urine.

These organs start participating, and because they have their own vibration—their own separate pulse that can be distinguished from the rest of the body—you start enhancing the total body response, whether it is the liver or the anatomic nervous system. Then add in nutrition and support for the detoxification pathways and all of sudden the body can work again. It's enabled itself once more. The body can start to finish its development, which often can be delayed or disrupted in such toxic bodies.

It wasn't as if the children weren't talking. It was more the fact that the body hadn't freed itself up enough to finish with its development. Toxins obviously took a priority. Development got the back seat. The innate intelligence in the body is so wise and concerned to keep you alive. Taking care of the toxins was more important than finishing up the development of speech. It was a life or death situation for the innate intelligence. The body needed to mobilize these toxins and move them to safer places. So it's the very act of the body's innate intelligence, deciding what to do with these toxins that stops development. And once you free up the bodies' stored toxins, and re-engage the pathways, the workload is less. The very development that was interrupted can start happening again. And that's definitely what I've seen.

David: Is there anything that we haven't talked about that you would like to add?

Leslie: I'd like to see moms back in the kitchen, controlling nutrition— again, from this perspective. It's part of the key to get back in the kitchen, to start cooking again—and not out of a box. It needs to be prepared properly. We've become such a fast-paced society that we've forgotten the value of a really well-cooked, nutritionally-dense meal— and what that does for the body. Properly grown foods offer the body an abundance of vitamins, enzymes, amino acids—all of that. In our home I use grass-fed beef, wild caught salmon, and organically grown produce. We drink raw milk from grass-fed cows. We eat a lot of raw ice cream. We sprout and soak organically-grown grains to make bread.

I avoid soy, processed sugar and genetically-modified foods. It is my personal quest, at this point to get moms back in the kitchen—re-inventing themselves, understanding the power of healing from within with foods. Chelation is a wonderful thing and it is necessary in today's times. But we've got to have a multi-approach attitude to this problem.

As a mom doing this, you feel quite isolated a lot of the time, and you are always second guessing yourself. The only thing that I ever had as a gauge was to look at the kids. I would often think, "They're acting better and more coherent, so there's got to be something that I'm doing right." Globally there were improvements. The kids are talking. I got eye contact this week. I'm happy.

I often tell people that my baby book is full of many first words, because sometimes you have language and sometimes you lose it. So the baby books are full and some people look at that as a problem. I look at that as a graciousness. I'm very grateful that there are many words, because there are still so many children who are not detoxing and who are silent. I think that's a tragedy.

Appendix C

An Interview with
Dr. Gerhard N. Schrauzer

By David Jay Brown

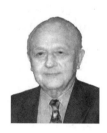 *Gerhard N. Schrauzer, Ph.D.—Professor Emeritus of Chemistry at the University of California, San Diego—is one of the world's experts on selenium and other nutritionally essential trace elements. He is internationally known and recognized for his work on the biological functions of vitamins and nutritionally essential trace elements—particularly selenium—and for his work on cancer prevention.*

Dr. Schrauzer received his Ph.D. in chemistry from the University of Munich in 1956. He is also a Certified Nutrition Specialist (CNS), and a Fellow of the American College of Nutrition (FACN), the American Association for Cancer Research, and other prestigious organizations. Dr. Schrauzer taught and carried out his research at UCSD from 1966 until 1994. In 1994 he founded the San Diego based Biological Trace Element Research Institute, which he presently directs.

Dr. Schrauzer's primary research interest involves cancer prevention, and the role that trace minerals and environmental toxins play in the disease. He has published more than three hundred research papers and reviews, has authored or edited four books—including Lithium in Biology and Medicine—*and he holds several U.S. patents. Dr. Schrauzer is also the Editor-in-Chief of the journal* Biological Trace Element Research, *a world-leading, peer-reviewed journal on the role of trace elements in biological systems.*

I interviewed Dr. Schrauzer on June 9, 2007. We spoke about the important role that selenium plays in the body, the benefits that an adequate daily dose of selenium provides, how selenium can be used to help detoxify the body from heavy metals, and how aging affects selenium levels in the body.

David: What originally inspired your interest in researching selenium?

Dr. Schrauzer: It arose from studies that we conducted that initially had very little to do with nutrition. We were interested in reactions involving the transfer of electrons between electron-donating sulfur compounds, such as thioglycerol, and acceptors like the organic dye methylene blue. We found this reduction to be catalyzed by selenium (in very small amounts), and it immediately struck me that this type of catalysis could be a biologically important because methylene blue—in terms of its behavior under reducing conditions—could be viewed as a analog of riboflavin (vitamin B2), and thioglycerol as a model for proteins or other biogenic compounds with sulfhydryl groups.

Oxidation-reduction reactions of proteins with sulfhydryl groups are part of the process of cellular respiration. Any disturbance of cellular respiration is dangerous as it could lead to the conversion of a normal cell into a cancer cell. A survey of the literature subsequently revealed that the same reaction had been used as a test in the 1950s to diagnose cancer at Massachusetts General Hospital and New York Medical College. This historical cancer test involved measuring the time it took for a certain amount of the methylene blue to be reduced in freshly drawn human plasma. The clinicians using this test noted that patients—among them often newly diagnosed patients with still microscopically small cancers—showed an inability to reduce methylene blue at significant rates. However, nobody knew why, until we demonstrated that it responded to the amount of selenium present in the plasma.

A positive test result thus showed that cancer patients had subnormal levels of selenium in their blood. This prompted studies with mice carrying a tumor virus which produces breast cancer in the females. We found that selenium significantly prevented the development of breast cancer in these mice. Thus, briefly, we got to selenium, from a simple chemical study to the recognition of selenium as nutritional anticarcinogenic agent.

David: Can you talk a little about the different forms of selenium and which form do you think should be used as a daily nutritional supplement?

Dr. Schrauzer: Selenium occurs in foods primarily as selenomethionine. Selenomethionine resembles methionine, a sulfur-containing amino acid, except that instead of sulfur it contains selenium. Major nutritional sources of selenomethionine are seafood (ocean fish such as tuna, etc.,) but also wheat, corn, rice, and soy—however, the latter only if they are grown in selenium-rich soil.

Since the consumption of seafood by Americans is rather low, and the selenium contents of the cereals are variable, selenium supplementation is the only sure way to achieve the desired two hundred to three hundred micrograms of selenium per day. For adults of average weight, a reasonable and safe supplemental dose of selenium is two hundred micrograms per day. The selenium should be in the form of selenomethionine. Strains of yeast cultivated in selenium-enriched media take up selenium and convert it naturally into selenomethionine. Supplements containing selenomethionine are available in health food stores.

Inorganic forms of selenium such as sodium selenite are also available and have some virtues, although they're not completely representing the natural nutritional situation because only selenomethionine can be significantly incorporated into proteins, thus allowing the selenium to be stored in the body. Ingested sodium selenite is used to produce the enzymes that contain selenium but this form of selenium cannot be stored.

David: What do you think is an adequate daily dosage of selenium for the average person to be taking?

Dr. Schrauzer: Our studies have demonstrated that the optimal dose for prevention purposes corresponds to approximately twice the average amount of selenium that Americans are currently getting—and that is between two hundred and maybe three hundred micrograms of selenium

per day. People on a normal American diet have selenium intakes ranging from around eighty to a hundred and fifty micrograms per day,
primarily because many areas of the United States are in fact selenium-
deficient.

Also, certain dietary habits cause us to obtain less selenium than we
should be getting. For example, if a significant percentage of your total
caloric intake comes from sugars and fats, both of which are virtually free
of essential trace minerals, then you are obviously not getting enough
selenium. Most people also do not realize that vegetables and fruit are
poor sources of selenium. The diets of vegetarians, while otherwise
healthy, often are selenium-deficient.

David: You mentioned seafood among the good nutritional sources of
selenium. But what about tuna, whose consumption we are to curtail
because of its mercury content?

Dr. Schrauzer: Apart from its selenium content, tuna is an excellent
source of protein and is also rich in omega-3 and omega-6 fatty acids.
There is no need to worry about the mercury present. The amounts are
small and, what is important, animals and humans effectively detoxify
mercury by combining it with selenium.

David: What are some of the benefits that an adequate daily dose of
selenium provides—especially with regard to treating heart disease,
cancer, and depression?

Dr. Schrauzer: Selenium is needed by all organs for optimal
function—including the heart, the brain, and the kidneys. Selenium is
a component of many enzymes, and more and more such enzymes are
being discovered. Our genome is actually specifically programmed to
produce these selenoenzymes. If we don't get enough selenium with our
diet these enzymes cannot be reproduced and the respective genes are
turned off. To offset the means of adaptation other genes are turned on.
As a result, our ability to withstand stress diminishes.

For example, our ability to withstand the damaging effects of aggressive
components in the atmosphere such as ozone diminishes because
selenium-dependent enzymes play a role in ozone detoxification. The

same enzymes, the glutathione S-transferases, also protect us from oxygen radicals that are produced under normal metabolic conditions. Oxygen radicals are reactive species which attack practically all organic cellular components. They can damage the DNA and cause mutations. To protect ourselves against oxygen radicals we must have enough selenium. That is one of the key functions of selenium in the human body, but there are many others—and some of them are in fact as yet unknown.

One group of enzymes are the so-called thioredoxin reductases. Thioredoxins are small peptides which contain sulfhydryl groups. These are used in the body to transfer electrons to where they're needed. In the process of their function, they are oxidized, and thus must be reduced first before they can do their job again. This is accomplished by the thioredoxin reductases.

Then we have the thyronine reductases. These enzymes are produced by, and mainly present in, the thyroid gland. Their primary function is to convert T4, the inactive precursor of the thyroid hormone into T3, its active form. Another, more recently discovered selenoenzyme, is Selenoprotein P. Its functions are not yet completely understood but it is believed to be mainly a selenium-transport protein.

David: How might selenium be helpful in detoxifying the body from heavy metals such as mercury?

Dr. Schrauzer: Selenium is nature's way to protect against mercury, and the previously mentioned Selenoprotein P is involved in this process. For example, people who had been occupationally exposed to mercury vapor were found to have high levels of mercury in their organs, especially in their brains, but they did not show signs of mercury toxicity. Their brains also contained high levels of selenium, which trapped the mercury in a nontoxic form.

David: Are there any health risks from too much selenium?

Dr. Schrauzer: The toxicity of selenium has been extensively studied. In fact, we know more about the toxicity of selenium than of practically any other element. According to current definitions by the Food and

Nutrition Board, three hundred and fifty micrograms of selenium per day represents the amount of selenium that is safe for an adult for indefinite periods. Another quantity is the NOAEL—or the 'No Adverse Effect Level'—which is eight hundred micrograms per day. The first symptoms of chronic toxicity appear after prolonged intakes of a thousand micrograms of selenium per day—prolonged meaning several months—and these symptoms are relatively harmless and reversible.

These levels are seldom reached under normal nutritional conditions and, as a result, supplemental selenium has an excellent safety record. Nonfatal cases of toxicity have occurred because of manufacturing errors, such as mistaking "mcg" (the symbol for micrograms) for "mg" (the symbol for milligrams), but only a few such cases have occurred during the past 30 years.

David: Is there a relationship between selenium and diabetes?

Dr. Schrauzer: Yes, in as much as studies have shown that selenium has a protective effect against diabetes. Recently some authors suggested that selenium somehow increased diabetes incidence in a group of subjects given selenium supplements, but the reasons for this may have been unrelated to selenium.

David: How does aging affect selenium levels in the body?

Dr. Schrauzer: As we age the absorption of selenium may decline, as is true for other nutrients. A study in a Japanese convalescent home demonstrated that the mortality was higher among residents with low serum selenium levels. A study in the United States showed the same to be true for elderly women. Since selenium is needed by all it is only logical to maintain a good selenium intake over one's entire life span.

David: Is there anything that we haven't spoke about that you would like to add?

Dr. Schrauzer: I would like reemphasize the importance of selenium for cancer prevention especially in light of the fact that some of the present dietary habits and fads such as, for example, the low carbohydrate diets, cause selenium intakes to decline. It should always be remembered that the old adage, a well balanced diet provides all vitamins and nutrients in adequate amounts, is not necessarily valid for selenium.

Appendix D

Chelation, Heavy Metals, Heart Disease, and Health: An Oral Detoxification Program That Is Now Essential for Optimal Health and Longevity

By Garry Gordon

This article originally appeared in the Townsend Letter for Doctors and Patients, *volume 287, June, 2007, pages 112-120.*

Introduction

At the recent Orthomolecular Medicine meeting in San Francisco, I mentioned to Dr. Jonathan Collin the tremendous success I was enjoying with our horses, using an oral protocol called the Oral Detoxification Program™ (ODP). My ODP protocol was dramatically improving the horses' performance beyond any expectations. Not long before, they had started competing in Grand Prix Jumping and had gone from being lame and tired and worth very little to jumping as high as five feet, five inches and becoming stars of the horse show. We collected 35 Blue Ribbons while competing against some 4,500 top show jumping horses at an annual Grand Prix Horse Show held in Thermal, California.

The horses were suddenly winning while competing against top jumpers, some of which are worth millions; most had trained rigorously for years. Our horses had only been on the ODP protocol for two to three months, and two had been quite lame three months before the show began. I had no idea that our rather nice but ordinary horses would suddenly come to life as they clearly did. Today, in fact, we now individualize their doses based on their show schedules. Grand Prix horse shows are generally won by the horse with the greatest endurance, so I "get their lead out." Today, many horses, like Barbaro, needlessly break legs. Until now, no one considers the level of lead and toxins in the bones of horses or humans. I intend to change that.

I have studied chelation therapy extensively, and in years past, I was director of a large Trace Element testing lab with offices in Amsterdam, Tokyo, and the San Francisco Bay area, testing lead, mercury, etc. in thousands of people from around the world. Despite those experiences, and despite reviewing thousands of articles I had collected and lectured about, I did not fully appreciate that the time had come to take action. Then, I was shocked into action by a series of photographs accompanying an October 2006 *National Geographic* article, "Chemicals Within Us."

Seeing the photographs of children with lead toxicity suddenly made me realize that, almost without exception, everyone is toxic today. If we are all to enjoy a higher level of health, we must start to routinely consume safe synergistic nutrients that can help us overcome these toxins. I came up with this idea for an advanced total nutritional detoxification protocol, using substances with which most of us have some familiarity, although we may not have seen the potential synergy achievable with the right combination. I made these nutrients into a comprehensive protocol that, with a few alterations, both my horses and my patients consume twice daily.

My own experience with IV chelation over 35 years ago changed my health dramatically; nonetheless, I never dreamed that similar powerful results would be possible with any oral-based protocol, so I did not really try. Since then, I have attempted to develop a program that simulates, for my patients, the benefits that I enjoyed after my first eight intravenous (IV) treatments were completed. I have continued to research this idea, spending a small fortune going to conferences around the world.

Over these years, I have participated in many other useful projects which include developing stabilized forms of vitamin C and Detox programs employing nutrients like stabilized rice bran. I worked with Dr. Lester Morrison on mucopolysaccharides. Using oral EDTA with mucopolysaccharides, I have been able to routinely lower blood viscosity as well as the incidence of fatal blood clots. These developments and many others came together finally in one protocol – ODP. (More details on the ODP protocol can be found on my website – www.gordonresearch. com – where various potential applications for this program, including those for pets, children, and adults are discussed in greater depth.)

Previously, I had employed many different treatments with which I had worked before, but I had never put it all together in one protocol. Once I could see how dramatically helpful this approach was with horses, I wanted to learn what it could do for many other athletes: either two- or four-legged. And, of course, all this has implications for anyone who just wants to optimize their health.

In the past, I had not considered using any form of chelation therapy for apparently well athletes. Now, it should be apparent that we have a widespread need for detoxification for everyone, not just athletes. Thus, the "walking wounded" who need to "get the lead out" will see results with my ODP protocol: longer lives, more energy, and less developing health problems. Today's levels of pollution have now made a life-long detoxification program beneficial for everyone, particularly if we want to achieve our maximum intended useful lifespan and enjoy optimal health. It seems obvious now that if IV chelation continues to help so many patients, we need a real Detox program for those who do not have the time, or finances, or who feel they need to wait until they are sick enough to qualify for IV chelation.

Once I realized that tired, lame horses could become champions, the thought crossed my mind that, yes, it might be fun to keep the details of our Blue-Ribbon-winning protocol a secret and have fun continuing to beat others in competition. I quickly decided that rather than just collecting more blue ribbons, I preferred to share what I have learned. As you read the rest of this article, I think you will agree that once the word gets out, my ODP protocol has the potential to change the face of athletic competition. I believe that ODP will raise the bar in all competitions so, to be competitive, everyone will need to be on effective long-term detoxification. Performance is easy to measure, whereas total body burdens of lead or mercury are complex and nearly impossible to accurately assess without costly test equipment, like that needed for the X-ray fluorescent measurement of bone offered at Harvard School of Public Health. I hope that this information will help others develop other even newer and more effective long-term strategies for lowering heavy metals in all living creatures.

Years ago, we lacked knowledge about long-term adverse effects of even very low levels of toxic heavy metals, such as we see in everyone today. We were also still learning about what we now see as the long-term safety of prolonged chelation. When I wrote the protocol for IV chelation for American College for Advancement in Medicine (ACAM), a process that took almost one year of my life, I had been warned that no deaths were ever to be attributed to my protocol. Thus I spent so much time satisfying that demand from the authorities that the wider potential applications of chelation therapy had to wait.

Now, we have had over ten million patients around the world with no known fatalities when my basic protocol was followed and proof that renal toxicity was almost non-existent. And, in fact, chelation therapy generally protects kidney function. Today, we have multiple published studies from mainstream medicine documenting the dangers of very low levels of lead and mercury. So, now is the time to begin to utilize this knowledge to improve the health of all living creatures. The potential benefits are finally becoming understood, and the risks are minimal compared to the benefits.

Years ago, I had to guard against giving the impression that chelation therapy in any form was some kind of a panacea for all health problems. Those of us treating documented severe heart disease patients met with tremendous resistance back then. I had been program chairman for ACAM when a leading expert on lead from Columbia University Medical School, who was my invited main speaker for an early ACAM conference and who was to speak on the adverse effects of lead on children, was researching DMSA. He stalked out of our conference after he heard the speaker before him, Dr. John Olwin, a vascular surgeon from Rush Medical College and a world-class expert on using IV ethylene diamine tetraacetic acid (EDTA) for vascular disease, state that lowering lead levels with IV EDTA would be helpful for cardiovascular disease. The expert refused to speak to our group, since he was only interested in studying lead toxicity for children. He was shocked that ACAM would permit someone to suggest that there was any connection between lead and cardiovascular disease. Now, we find lead to be a "Silent Killer," so-called in 2006 in *Circulation*, the voice of the American Heart Association. Until recently, chelating doctors have focused on chelation therapy primarily for severe heavy metal poisoning or for vascular disease.

Moving Beyond Simple Cardiovascular Care

I have lectured around the world about the massive increases of lead and mercury building up in all living things for many years. There is extensively published literature today that clearly documents that getting the lead out is crucial for optimal health (Nawrot TS. Low-level environmental exposure to lead unmasked as silent killer. *Circulation*. 2006; 114: 1347-1349). I am convinced that my ODP protocol, along with IV chelation, can safely cancel nearly 90% of heart bypass and stenting operations for coronary arteriosclerosis. We need to begin to use the ODP protocol for far broader, non–cardiovascular-related applications. We should no longer focus on simply preventing heart attacks.

We all need more energy and better memories, and we no longer need to base the decision on whether or not to treat on how advanced our occlusive vascular disease has become. Today, for instance, one in four children is prescribed drugs for everything from ADHD to autism, depression, diabetes, or cancer. We need to start treating at the preconception level and help eliminate illnesses in children. Detoxifying children at all ages will lead to improved performance in sports or scholastics. As this improvement becomes widely known, others will become more interested in lowering the level of toxins in their bodies. In turn, this might lead to a greater demand for cleaner water, food, and air.

Over the past 20 years, I have received hundreds of testimonials from clients around the world who report many benefits from what I previously categorized as a form of oral chelation. However, the term oral chelation has become so abused that we may need to drop it. We have autistic children who need heavy metal detox and heart disease patients unsure if they need chelation therapy or just some oral program. Those who need their mercury and lead levels lowered have no idea what really works and what is hype. They are confused about where to turn and what to do, so many wind up doing nothing. Patients are told by some doctors that orally ingested EDTA is worthless; while other doctors suggest that taking oral EDTA is such a great approach that, particularly if administered with liposome or taken rectally or topically, no one ever needs IV chelation.

Today, we can often benefit cardiovascular patients, sometimes dramatically, even without any form of chelation therapy. No one can fail to appreciate the importance of recent, often dramatic new developments in nutrition: supplementation with ribose, lipoic acid, co-enzyme Q-10, carnitine, magnesium, garlic, vitamin K-2, vitamin C, stabilized rice bran, omega 3, Wobenzym®, resveratrol, etc. The documented benefits from these and other advanced nutrient therapies are changing nutritional medicine and have led to a new field called metabolic cardiology.

Some of these developments can eliminate the need for pharmaceutical therapy. For example, we now recognize that most people do not get enough minerals such as selenium or magnesium, nor do they receive enough fiber or vitamins C, E, D, or K. Some so-called oral chelation programs simply employ certain nutritional concepts that may improve heavy metal excretion, but do not offer adequate nutritional support to really help lower overall morbidity and mortality from heart attacks and strokes. Other so-called oral chelation programs just employ a few herbs and provide little hope for any real long-term benefit to the user, often at high price, claiming miraculous overnight removal of all toxic metals, which is clearly not possible.

I think that the most potentially harmful aspect of these poorly formulated products is that they can further confuse consumers who soon find that those products do little or nothing – and who then turn to drugs to help deal with their health issues. In contrast, with an adequate explanation of what to expect along with my ODP protocol, patients will be warned not to expect overnight miracles. This way many may stay with the protocol long enough to really see their symptoms abate and their need for drug-based therapies substantially reduced over time. Everyone today has numerous neurotoxins and carcinogens in their blood at all times, and the longer they follow my ODP protocol, the lower all toxin levels will become and the better they will feel.

No one can really provide significant long-term detox benefits over a lifetime by simply using a single chelator, whether that is EDTA, DMSA, malic acid, or ascorbic acid, delivered by any route – inhaled, used topically or rectally, or liposome-treated, for a few weeks or even a couple of years. We now live on a toxic planet, and, if you stop my detox program, heavy metals will reaccumulate, and you cannot eliminate much of your body burden of toxins overnight. Short-term treatment can be very useful and may stop angina and or offer often-dramatic symptomatic relief, but I like to think in terms of no more heart attacks for the next 20-plus years. We are all living longer, now let's live better.

My early oral chelation protocol, Beyond Chelation, routinely helped eliminate most symptoms of advancing cardiovascular problems. I believe many of the benefits seen were largely due to Dr. Morrison's mucopolysaccharide/EDTA contribution. His research developed a safe nutritional program that routinely lowers blood viscosity to the level seen in menstruating females, who, incidentally, seldom have fatal heart attacks. We now understand how blood viscosity and circulatory health are related.

Since my ODP protocol predictably eliminates most heart attacks and strokes, you may then focus on other goals, such as helping your patients avoid health problems associated with aging, such as Alzheimer's disease, cancer, osteoporosis, etc. I believe my earlier basic protocol of Beyond Chelation (and later, Beyond Chelation Improved), has added many years to patients' lives around the world. If you are planning to live into your 80s, the added protection from my far more comprehensive ODP protocol will make sense. Clearly, we are all living longer, and the Alzheimer's Foundation predicts that by age 85, 50% of patients will have Alzheimer's disease. I am unaware of any of my patients developing Alzheimer's disease in the past 20-plus years. This is not just due to lower blood viscosity or lower lead levels that Beyond Chelation Improved produces, but Beyond Chelation has always included ingredients like Phosphatidylserine and Ginkgo Biloba, which have been a routine part of my oral protocol for over 20 years now. All my patients are instructed to take their nine-pill packets twice a day.

Recently, I have worked with autistic children and have successfully co-developed a protocol getting mercury out of all children, without exception even when IV chelation previously had produced little or no effect. Sometimes we find excretion levels off the chart at Doctors Data lab on urine and or feces. This heavy excretion sometimes continues for more than six months to two years. This "autism" program does not require the use of IV therapies. I mention these applications to show that we are all still learning about heavy metals and their removal. We need to keep open minds about which treatments will eventually become widely adopted and which, over time, should fall by the wayside.

Building an Open Dialogue and Sharing Information

Although it is still too early to lay down any hard and fast rules, hopefully, we can begin an open dialogue. I now have over 1,100 physicians as members of my Forum on Anti-Aging and Chelation Therapy (FACT) online discussion group. All licensed health professionals are invited to join and search on our site for comments from the group on any topic from DMPS to Lipoic acid to autism. You are encouraged to offer your observations and comments if you join the FACT group. (Applications may be made at www.gordonresearch.com.) In addition, I created a special area on my website (www. gordonresearch.com/townsend) to support the comments in this article and further this discussion. There you can find many articles I refer to here, and also the *National Geographic* photographs, which you can review and download.

I have written more about the mechanisms of action of EDTA than any other researcher/author in the world, yet I know that we still lack adequate knowledge to maximize all the potential benefits. We will need to learn more as our world becomes increasingly toxic. Most experts agree today that there is no safe level of lead or mercury. I am totally convinced of the long-term safety and minimal risk from continual administration of these metal-binding substances or chelators, including malic acid, garlic, DMSA, EDTA, ascorbic acid, and even fiber. The alternative, to just live with these toxins, is no longer feasible. I have decided to vigorously promote the use of chelators all over the world. Once you review some of the over 500 articles I have selected from the over 7,000 articles written on just EDTA over the past 35 years, you can better decide if you want to personally choose an ODP protocol for yourself and/or your family.

As one of the major early proponents introducing IV chelation therapy to the world over the past 35 years, I have had to defend myself from medical society challenges and medical boards' litigation. Therefore, I have amassed an extensive library on the subject. I want to share as much of that information with you here and on my website as possible.

For your convenience, I have placed 500 abstracts on oral EDTA on my website (www.gordonresearch.com), where use of the available Search feature will help provide easy access to information that may change your life, as it has mine. Just use any word, such as lead, mercury, EDTA, DMSA, malic acid, or garlic etc. Then you will conveniently access some of the scientific information that I have collected over the past 30-plus years since I co-founded what became known as ACAM.

I also have developed over my nearly 50 years of medical practice many in-depth protocols for treating various conditions like cancer, multiple sclerosis, ALS, Parkinson's, Alzheimer's, etc. Those may only be accessed by joining FACT, which, as noted earlier, is only for licensed health professionals. Currently, over 1,100 health professional members tell me they find this discussion group invaluable. Members can query FACT on any subject and often quickly get help from colleagues. FACT works as an open and searchable "curbside consultation" from colleagues on almost any health-related topic. Access to FACT requires registration. Members are then assigned a password that will permit them to read daily updates, ask questions or search my protocols on many topics from autism to prostate cancer, etc.

Practitioners will enjoy the many positive comments there from the many leading chelation doctors who have started to incorporate some new ideas they picked up on this site. For example, many seem interested to share results they are seeing in patients after they finally try the short chelation, particularly after years of offering only the three-hour version of IV chelation. Many comment that this approach permits them to offer help to patients who could not arrange the necessary time from work or finances for the longer form. Most seem to feel that the shorter IV helps more patients faster, no matter what the diagnosis.

Medical progress often means that things we previously believed may no longer be true. I know that many ideas that I expressed over 30 years ago in writing and teaching about chelation therapy were simply wrong, like my belief in the early years that we had found a magic "roto-rooter" that routinely diminished plaque on arteries. Clearly, I was wrong, and that concept is no longer valid. Many chelating doctors, including those at ACAM, were initially worried about using my short chelation employing IV calcium EDTA. In particular, they argued that if the patient's vessels are already calcified, IV calcium was contraindicated, but, in fact, the truth seems to be that high transient levels of IV-administered calcium can actually provide many beneficial actions in the body. If lowering lead levels is as important as many experts now believe, then clearly calcium EDTA, which is routinely extracting more lead than the slow infusions of sodium EDTA, may wind up becoming the treatment of choice for many patients.

Doctors using the FACT website generally report better results than they were seeing with the three-hour treatment, which many have used for 20 years. Of course, many doctors using FACT have learned more about my other detoxification programs and now employ the broader protocol: my ODP protocol. There are many added components here; in its simplest form, the protocol adds the proprietary form of well-tolerated and better-absorbed vitamin C complex called Bio En'R-G'y and the Advanced Beyond Fiber with inulin and stabilized rice bran. When these are employed, along with metal-binding nutrients, then you have the basis of my ODP protocol.

I believe that the doctors using this broader protocol may skew the results reported by the 1100 doctors using the FACT discussion group. Since we all have better nutritional support programs for our patients, the IV EDTA is no longer the main active component in our therapy. With the new short form of Calcium EDTA, our IV chelation efforts are more focused on what I believe should be its primary function, which is mainly enhancing lead and heavy metal excretion. This may lead you, as a practicing health professional, to see that, from the first visit on, this advanced ODP protocol is protecting your patients more than ten chelation treatments would, because of the vastly improved total protocol, particularly with the oral heparin-like activity we provide, virtually eliminating the formation of pathologic blood clots.

In addition, most chelating doctors today know much more about heart disease and nutritional approaches to heart disease treatment than we knew 35 years ago back in the infancy of the chelation movement. I believe that most of us now routinely use a more sophisticated and broader spectrum in their management of their cardiovascular patients – indeed, all their patients. Many of their patients today with cardiovascular disease are receiving far superior nutritional support to anything we dreamed about 35 years ago when I wrote, for ACAM, that first protocol for safe use of IV EDTA in vascular disease. When I wrote that protocol, I was strongly motivated by the demand of the State of California authorities who said in essence, "develop a protocol or we will stop all further chelation by members of your group." Today, many of us are incorporating the new well-documented menaquinone-7 form of K-2 along with programs using at least some of the elements of my ODP protocol in treating calcified coronaries.

The ODP Protocol Response: Getting the Lead Out

My basic ODP protocol involves special combinations of stabilized fiber, combined with an advanced form of stabilized vitamin C and calcium EDTA. The horses clearly have responded beyond my wildest dreams to this simple ODP protocol. I think that since athletes no longer can legally continue to abuse their bodies with drugs, many of them may want to learn about the dramatic benefits they can enjoy from this legal detox protocol that I am convinced will help any athlete, at any age, perform better. Of course, those who are on my ODP protocol will start to raise the bar for all other athletes. Those not on an effective protocol that really is getting the lead out will truly be competing with a handicap. This applies equally to scholastic performance at all levels including spelling or math competitions for children. It is documented, by the Centers for Disease Control and the Environmental Protection Agency, that the higher the lead, the lower the IQ, the energy level, and even lifetime earnings potential will be. Programs like ODP can help keep our country more competitive in world markets, since when our work force is healthier, we are more competitive.

We know there are probably thousands of toxins adversely affecting us, and my protocol helps deal with many of them, but focusing on lead and mercury helps to simplify our understanding regarding why this is a marathon, not a sprint. This is a lifetime project. Lead is primarily concentrated in bones, where it is not readily assessable to chelation. There are no chelators or detox programs that, contrary to wild claims being made, can significantly access our average thousandfold increase in bone lead stores in the one to three months most programs are claiming. Any real treatment must be continued long enough for bones to completely remodel. For children, this is five-plus years, for adults,

15-plus years.

The surprisingly dramatic responses from detoxing our horses reminded me that over 15 years ago, a top racehorse vet in Canada attended an ACAM conference where I was in charge, and he gave me his book. He explained to attendees from the podium that he regularly chelated his clients' horses intravenously. Like most doctors today, back then I was only focused on the cardiovascular and circulatory benefits from IV chelation, never thinking that in time pollution would become so serious that we would all need a lifetime gentle detoxification protocol. Now, low-level lead levels are adversely affecting everything, including the cardiovascular system, thus removing lead alone could explain some of the often rather dramatic improvements seen in chelated patients who may clinically improve (again, often dramatically), but who, all too often, may not have enjoyed any reversal in obstructing areas of plaque.

I initially focused on trying to reduce obstructing plaques, believing that the limiting blood flow to crucial areas is the main reason for symptoms. Yet, over the years we now know that we can restore most heart patients to apparent high-level cardiovascular status with IV EDTA chelation therapy and yet often find there is no accompanying reduction in plaque; in some cases, plaque even becomes worse, even when the patient takes 30 or more IV chelation treatments. I have explained several reasons for this paradox in prior articles, where I list over 30 possible mechanisms of action for IV EDTA chelation. One small example from that list is that improved nitric oxide metabolism associated with getting the "lead out" can dramatically improve endurance and blood flow.

Over the years, I have been consulted routinely about patients whose coronary calcium levels soar while on IV or oral chelation. As mentioned, we have seen plaque become even more obstructive, yet often the patient may have become symptom-free in spite of this clear-cut worsening of their case technically. This indicates to me that IV chelation does not predictably routinely reverse coronary arteriosclerosis, but getting the "lead out" with IV chelation or with my ODP protocol may be just as or even more important than reversing plaque. The optimal solution is not either IV or oral; the answer is both.

Today, with ultra hi-speed coronary cat scans, we have an easy measurement for coronary vessel calcium levels, so more patients can now be treated more adequately on a preventive basis and will come to realize that detoxification is a life-long protocol. My ODP protocol now also electively incorporates therapeutic levels of vitamin K-2 and more recently, the Herbal Remedy from Thailand (HRT; actual technical name is Pueraria Mirifica), which is a bio-mimic estrogenic adaptogen, to enhance the desired effects of calcium relocation whenever significant vascular calcification is documented. My complete protocol routinely lowers pathologic calcium in coronary arteries, while reversing osteoporosis.

I believe that ODP will, over time, provide highly effective symptomatic improvement in well over 80% of patients, particularly now that we have ancillary approaches with diet, exercise, the new fibrin-digesting and anti-inflammatory enzymes, and useful supplements like ribose, lipoic acid, resveratrol, co-enzyme Q-10, etc. Any or all of those can be added to the basic protocol, so that, with all these additional well-documented nutrients available to us today for cardiovascular disease, I seldom fail to achieve the response my patient seeks. I have often cancelled recommended heart transplants in children and adults because the response has been so good.

The benefits seen with my ODP protocol alone are not achieved as rapidly as IV chelation results may be. I would not expect the ODP protocol to provide the dramatic increase in endurance that IV chelation gave me. By my eighth IV (over a three-week interval), my disabling angina was completely gone. At that point, and for the first time in years, I also had no dyspnea on exertion. I could run up a mountain and wear out my two-year-old Irish Setter. My response was so dramatic that I have devoted the past 35 years to trying to learn how and why IV chelation provides these effects in some patients. I believe that with my protocol, we can now start to deliver some of those benefits to millions around the world who simply want to get the "lead out" and start to enjoy a far higher level of health.

Chelation Choices

Now, since I believe we have these choices, when do we absolutely need IV chelation? That decision must remain in the hands of the physician. It never hurts to do both, but I argue here that I do not believe IV chelation alone is ever enough. If we are to really stop most fatal heart attacks, we need long-term daily protection. I believe nothing currently available today exceeds the efficacy I achieve with my patients on my ODP protocol.

Clearly, when a patient calls about an acute condition, such as the recent onset of stroke or pulmonary embolism or heart attack, I have always explained that, ideally, IV chelation should be started as soon as possible. Meantime, however, we can use oral enzymes including Wobenzym®, Nattokinase, and/or Boluoke®. These enzymes can, in my estimation, save lives. Tissue Plasminogen Activator (tPA) was the first to show that clots could be dissolved after they form. Tissue Plasminogen Activator is rather expensive, must be given through an IV in a hospital environment, and has a very narrow window of opportunity with which to work. It has been proven useful for dissolving fresh blood clots. Nattokinase and Lumbrokinase (Boluoke®) offer similar effects, but I prefer to take them preventively, although there have been reports of favorable effects even days after the stroke or heart attack, often using double doses of these oral preparations, which may be more effective in some cases than the IV injection of tPA.

These enzymes and other therapies like Hyperbaric Oxygen (HBO) therapy and IV chelation offer surprising benefits, even a few days after a major circulatory event. Oral enzyme products may provide some fibrin-digesting activity and anti-inflammatory activity. They can be used along with Essential Daily Defense, the key product resulting from Dr. Morrison's research. Essential Daily Defense is a crucial part of the ODP protocol. It offers a gentle but vital heparin-like effect that I believe significantly contributes to my remarkable success preventing any reported fatal MIs in users of my ODP protocol. I always recommend that patients with any acute condition also get IV treatments, even IV magnesium, and/or ascorbic acid can offer huge benefits if EDTA is not available. This IV can be administered as either the new short form of IV chelation or the standard version or given one after the other, as an

IV Myers Cocktail after an IV chelation treatment.

Generally, IV Chelation therapy always will work quicker, and perhaps cleanse deeper, as Simonizing does more than just wash a car. IV EDTA generally, in one day, removes as much lead as two to three weeks of oral chelating. This enhanced lead excretion seems to be particularly true with the new short form of chelating that I have recently helped introduce to the world. This IV uses calcium EDTA. This form of EDTA treatment is entirely painless and thus can be conveniently given in five 15 minute sessions, saving patients valuable time and money. The more rapid infusion time means that blood levels of EDTA will be higher. I have also found that the short form of IV chelation routinely removes more lead per treatment than we see with the three-hour standard chelation.

There will probably be some continuing need for the original three-hour IV chelation treatment for many years. We now believe that protocol has helped over 10 million patients worldwide without a single known fatality. That protocol, which I initially wrote for ACAM over 35 years ago, has proven itself, and there is no need for it to be replaced. However, I always look for ways to make other people feel as good as I do, having had only four IV chelations in the past 15 years, after needing nearly 200 IV chelations prior to that, but not going a day without some oral chelation every 12 hours for the past 20-plus years. Now with the increasing mercury levels in our environment, I have increased my personal program and have added daily Heavy Detox (with DMSA).

Treating Vascular Calcifications

Most doctors are more familiar and therefore more comfortable with the original IV Chelation therapy. There is no right or wrong answer regarding who needs the shorter treatment and who needs the longer, older treatment. However, recently, the three-hour form of chelation technically has become slightly less necessary, since it appears that vascular calcifications are routinely reversible with advanced targeted nutritional support therapy that includes vitamin K-2 (menaquinone-7), which by itself routinely lowers pathologic calcium in vascular tissue. Nonetheless, I also prefer to increase bone health at the same time as I lower vascular calcium levels.

There was a time when patients with vascular calcification had to hope that the three-hour IV EDTA treatment would treat their problem. This was because the IV EDTA three-hour treatment lowers serum calcium levels, often by 50%, and therefore induces a tripling of Parathormone (PTH) production. This spurt of PTH theoretically should help lower pathologic calcium levels in many tissues. I have studied the subject of pathological calcium increases associated with aging of our vascular tissues extensively for many years. We all get calcified vascular tissues the older we are. The average aorta at age 80 contains 140 times more calcium than at age ten.

Calcified vascular tissue is a proven risk factor for heart disease. One problem is that it contributes to stiffness and loss of elasticity, thereby increasing the workload for the heart. This may contribute to rising blood pressure along with other factors. I now routinely expect to reverse both osteoporosis and vascular calcifications with newer approaches I have developed. Herbal Remedy from Thailand and vitamin K-2 (which I formulated into a synergistic formula, Beyond Bone Defense) with strontium, boron, curcumin, and other factors, has worked very well on everyone so far. I treat the bones and the vascular tissues concurrently, since I believe that as we prevent and reverse osteoporosis, there will be less vascular calcification. Since lead contributes to bone-related issues, I also incorporate my ODP-based approach with the above.

Beyond Chelation Improved

A key part of my ODP protocol is called Beyond Chelation Improved. This product contains nine pills in one convenient cellophane packet, which is usually taken twice a day. I co-developed the Beyond Chelation Improved formula more than 20 years ago with Dr. Lester Morrison. Three capsules in each packet of nine pills form the key part of the formula called Essential Daily Defense. This contains a unique heparin-like mucopolysaccharide from red algae, identified by Dr. Morrison (after ten million dollars in research), as an agent for reversing and preventing arteriosclerosis.

I was in radiology in 1964 in San Francisco at Mount Zion Hospital, because my disabling angina onset at age 29 forced me to close my general practice and go into residency. Since then, I have actively studied the benefit-risk ratio for most therapies offered to cardiovascular patients. Remember most fatal MIs are due to acute blood clots. Clots do not easily form in the presence of heparin. There is a gentle, safe anticoagulant effect with our combination of EDTA when in the presence of the particular mucopolysaccharide that I have found can replace injections of heparin for life-long protection.

Dr. Morrison's goal was to lower clotting tendencies. I find this formula reduces the need for aspirin-related therapies, since it works as he intended and described in detail in the three books that summarize his years of research in solving this problem. I often find that with this product as a vital part of my anti-clotting protocol, along with many other things including omega 3 supplementation, etc., I am able to routinely offer effective all-natural, anti-clotting, anti-platelet approaches for my patients who often do not tolerate drugs like Plavix® or Coumadin®. However, my patients are warned that they must assume full responsibility if they decide to discontinue their Coumadin®.

I will, whenever possible, urge that they also take the Nattokinase or Boluoke; however, due to cost, some have to rely on just the protection provided by the old standby, Beyond Chelation Improved. If possible, I prefer patients stay on my more comprehensive ODP protocol where the unique stabilized vitamin C and Beyond Fiber add so much. And, of course, enzymes – like Wobenzym, or those with Nattokinase, such as Endokinase, or Lumbrokinase, (Boluoke) – whether used alone or together in low doses, provide optimal protection, which, in my opinion, vastly exceeds the benefits from Plavix® or Coumadin® and related drugs.

Beyond Chelation Improved also includes three tablets of Beyond Any Multiple, so that all mineral and vitamin needs are included in the packet. I find few formulas exceed the total nutrients in this therapeutic strength multiple, which is another key part of my ODP protocol. Because our increasing levels of chronic toxicity also increase the need for many nutrients, this formula contains things like resveratrol, beta glucan, and lipoic acid, as well as things like high levels of vitamin D, selenium, and ultra trace minerals like cesium. Since there are many toxins, such as the residual toxins from ever-present flame retardants in all of us today that nothing can effectively deal with, I believe that to minimize the danger, we should always provide broad-spectrum, super-nutritional support. That is because a better nourished body can tolerate these often still poorly identified toxic reactions, like chronic neurotoxicity and carcinogenic potential from the usual array of over 100 organic toxins documented to be present in virtually all humans today.

Understanding Chelation and Lifetime Detoxification

Like many of you, I still offer IV chelation to my patients. I love to observe the often dramatic improvement we sometimes see in our IV-treated patients. Obviously with patients with recent stroke or gangrene, I will also use everything from HBO to IV chelation and Nattokinase or Boluoke and Wobenzym. But, I fear that due to confusion and lack of knowledge about what was loosely called oral chelation, the end result of this confusion is that most of us today fail to recommend enough oral chelators for our patients. It seems that some practitioners are afraid to add to the confusion. In the consumer's mind, it's either one form of chelation or the other.

This confusion means that many doctors fail to effectively lower blood viscosity or provide safe anti-coagulants over a lifetime. Far too few patients understand – unless someone educates them on the long-term implications of today's pollution and the need for continued lifetime detoxification – that although all their symptoms may have disappeared, they can still have a massive MI at anytime – unless they make use of the substantial protection offered by the ODP protocol. My ODP concept goes beyond providing another oral chelation product. It is meant to help us all focus more on our vital need for long-term detoxification, and I hope this concept will help many more patients receive optimal treatment.

Remember the tortoise and the hare? You won't necessarily win the race by the speed with which you improve your patients' conditions; the real race will be won when your patients understand the long-term view, when you inform them what your protocol can and cannot do, and when they understand how vital it is that they never stop their oral protocol. I am now convinced that the Beyond Chelation Improved formula was a very important breakthrough in medicine. In 1941, Dr. Morrison published his research on cholesterol in the *Journal of American Medical Association*

(JAMA), but he almost immediately concluded that cholesterol was not the main culprit. He then went to work on researching clotting and blood viscosity. This I am convinced is where the future lies, and in a few years, we will see that statins have been an expensive experiment for our country. Statins cause provable harm and provide little benefit compared to the protocol I have developed.

Certainly, they will not cause horses to win blue ribbons. We have many reasons to explain why we generally find today, after adequate testing, that our patients tend to be hypercoagulable, particularly at the time they suffer their acute MI or stroke. The reasons are complex and include genetics (five percent of Americans have LEIDEN 5 as a risk factor), stress, chronic infections, and heightened levels of toxins. I believe that, today, combating this clot-forming tendency has become essential for long-term survival for the majority of patients. I consider aspirin to be totally inadequate and the benefit-to-risk ratio causes me to not bother using it. Also, taking aspirin provides a false sense of security; and since patients do not realize how little protection it provides them, consequently, they do not bother to look further and find out about programs like my ODP protocol, which really provides clear-cut, long-term benefits with no downside.

I am convinced that the total ODP protocol, particularly if I add either Boluoke or Nattokinase, will result in far fewer deaths and/or need for any subsequent hospitalization or surgical intervention than any protocol currently offered anywhere else in the world. I routinely advise my patients against most invasive procedures for coronary artery disease, since I am convinced they all carry significantly greater risk than my approach. There are many complex reasons for the success of my protocol. I am sure I have not yet fully identified all of them. With over 100 active ingredients in the total protocol, the complex synergies at work will not be easy to separate and study.

Those too busy to learn about the ten million dollars that went into the formula might misconstrue Beyond Chelation Improved as just another oral chelation product. The Beyond Chelation Improved product is clearly far more complex than the oral or rectal administration of EDTA or the application of DMSA or DMPS on the skin. Those approaches are clearly inadequate when you realize the minimum 15-year requirement for ongoing therapy. I hope my ODP concept helps us move beyond the confusion that an imprecision of terms has contributed to this ongoing IV vs. oral chelation therapy controversy.

There are antioxidant benefits from several of the oral chelators in my ODP formula. I would expect my protocol will lead to improved energy and vitality, which, over time, may also help lower the total body burden of pathogens. With detoxification, enhanced immunity will follow. That alone helps control the level of pathogens. However, with any ill patients, to lower their total pathogen burden dramatically, some oxidative therapies should be considered.

I am confident taking my new ODP complete protocol daily for life provides greater protection against sudden death than 50 IV chelation treatments taken over one to three years, which is too short a time for long-term benefit to develop. Experts agree that the oral EDTA, which is a small part of the ODP protocol, has only about five percent to 18% absorption rates. This is a vital component in providing the heparin-life effect we need. Remember that there are only a few drops in the bottom of a lavender tube for a CBC, but that is all it takes to prevent those blood specimens from clotting.

The protocol also lowers lead levels slowly, continuously, over their entire lifetime if they choose to follow my ODP protocol. However, I do not believe that being lead-free or mercury-free is enough to prevent fatal blood clots. My ODP protocol involves much more. However, we have many other reasons to focus on safe long-term lead and mercury detoxification. Those references relate to IQ and worker productivity over time, as well as lower lead levels' link to lowering all causes of morbidity and mortality. The *New England Journal of Medicine* (NEJM) published research stating that calcium EDTA reduces the likelihood of renal failure as well as the subsequent need for dialysis. A Harvard School of Public Health study, published in *JAMA* a year ago, links cataract development to the level of lead in bones. This shows bone lead is in equilibrium with all tissues, including the lens of the eye.

The multiple health benefits from toxic metal removal achievable with my new ODP protocol seem to continue to increase the longer the protocol is continued. However, even after seven years on this protocol, adults still will have lowered their bone lead levels by only 50%. Dr. Clair Patterson from Cal Tech has spoken at ACAM twice at my invitation. His impressive world-wide research has proven that average bone lead levels today are well over 1,000 times higher than bone lead levels were just 400 years ago, anywhere you live on earth today. There is no escape, but after seven years with my nonstop protocol, you should have only 500 times too much lead still remaining, which still can help kill you if you become injured and inactive.

Remember, inactivity accelerates osteoporosis. This accelerates the loss of bone lead and its subsequent increase in your other tissues, impairing immunity, leaving you vulnerable to hospital-acquired infections. That is a hidden benefit of becoming as lead-free as possible. After 15 years, you will be much less likely to die of complications should you inadvertently wind up in a hospital.

Pro-Oxidative Therapies

I have given many lectures on pro-oxidative therapies, a vital adjunct to detoxification. Nothing else deals as effectively with the pathogen burden. You may view more on these topics online at http://www. gordonresearch.com/category_presentations.html. You can also view the entire proceedings from my highly successful, exciting March 10, 2007 conference. If you have a patient suffering from cancer and all else is failing, please watch the Dr. Contreras presentation.

Dr. Contreras documents how to administer oxygen therapies with high-dose IV vitamin C. Vitamin C alone will not work, as cancer cells are hypoxic and the vitamin C must be metabolized intracellular into H_2O_2. He documents substantial benefits using this protocol, after all chemo and radiation and all other alternative cancer therapies have failed. I have been teaching the methods and reasons for alternating between high-dose, pro-oxidant therapy and my new ultimate form of vitamin C (Bio En'R-G'y C) for truly effective, life-long antioxidant therapy. Since the recent *JAMA* article alleging that antioxidants are harmful, the study of pro-oxidant and antioxidant therapies is vital; we owe it to ourselves and our patients to understand the genesis of the *JAMA* article's confusion.

I am excited to have co-developed a professional version of vitamin C that is proven to provide benefits that no form of vitamin C has ever provided before. Bio En'R-G'y C with GMS-Ribose is also uniquely tolerated in very high doses without gastrointestinal (GI) upset. This formula has been documented to lower Reactive Oxygen Species at ppb levels, a benefit never achieved before with any vitamin C product in the world. Clearly, Bio En'R-G'Y C is a nutrient system and not just a vitamin C.

Dr. Contreras's research with pro-oxidant therapy documents significant life prolongation and tumor reduction in over 90% of terminal cancer patients with his IV vitamin C and oxygen in a new protocol with Perftec. Yet clearly, we do not want high-level pro-oxidant activity every day of our lives, so now we can safely cycle back to effective antioxidants, based on this new stabilized form of oral Bio En'R-G'y C formula.

In general, vitamin C, like all weak organic acids, is also a chelator, thus workers in lead factories taking vitamin C orally have lower levels of lead than those not taking it. This means that high-dose IV ascorbic acid is working both as a pro-oxidant therapy and a chelator. I believe that learning more about the benefits and risks of aggressive high-dose IV vitamin C treatment may save lots of lives, since such treatment combines at least those two vital functions at once. It can lower heavy metal levels while also lowering the total body burden of pathogens and tumor cells. I almost always prefer to augment that chelation effect with EDTA and my oral ODP protocol.

I hope you will come to future ACAM conferences and learn more about oxidative therapies, since we all face cancer or antibiotic-resistant infections such as Lyme disease, etc., everyday. I find that oxidative therapies can offer a realistic solution to antibiotic-resistant infections and, with the coming epidemics of infections experts predict, you will need this new information.

We need to learn how to maximize, for the majority of our lives, effective antioxidant therapies, which we can enhance with concurrent administration of some nutritional metal-binding agents or oral chelators. Some oral chelators may increase the antioxidant effect of other nutrients, while concurrently helping to lower levels of heavy metals at the same time. They may even help stabilize other useful nutrients, such as vitamin C, which, in the presence of the metal-binding agents I have selected, may finally turn out to be even more useful than Linus Pauling predicted. Vitamin C could, with the help of some oral chelators, turn out to be the ideal oral chelator, universal antioxidant, and all-purpose nutrient support molecule that we all have hoped it would be.

Nutritional Chelators: Supporting Nutrition While Removing Toxic Metals

The need for improved nutrition is just one side of the coin in bettering health. We get more benefits from nutritional support, however, when we also deal with heavy metal toxicity. Since we now know we cannot hope to get all the toxic metals out in less than a few years, we should always be concurrently improving total nutritional intake. This approach permits the body to function better during the many months and years needed to lower the levels of toxic metals. Fortunately, we do not need to remove all heavy metals to function much better; the correct combinations of natural nutritional chelators can bind toxic metals so that their adverse effects on health is almost eliminated temporarily, that is, as long as nutritional chelators are continued and practitioners start to learn the whole story on metal-binding and treat patients for the long-term, not just the short-term.

The Oral Detoxification Program: A Wide-Spectrum Protocol

Certain natural chelators can also be powerful antioxidants, but there is no single chelator that can meet all the needs of various tissues to bind different metals with different valences under different conditions of oxygen availability and differing pH levels. That is why I like my broadly based new program, the Oral Detoxification Protocol (ODP), which I am using on my patients and my horses. [See Part One of this article in the June issue of *Townsend Letter* for a complete introduction to my ODP.] With ODP, I am not relying on just one substance to lower the activity of metal-induced free radical mediated reactions.

It's important that patients always take the ODP with its high-potency supplements. To make that unavoidable, I have had the basic program that started all this, the Beyond Chelation Improved, combined into a nine-pill packet. This means that every one of my patients always receives Omega 3 supplementation and primrose oil and a high-potency multiple. I cannot risk anyone ever becoming mineral-depleted with my long-term ODP, although the evidence is that some of the so-called chelators employed may actually enhance the availability of some minerals, such as cobalt, rather than always depleting them, contrary to popular belief about long-term ingestion of metal-binding agents. For the past 20 years, I haven't gone anywhere without my total ODP. Lately, I have begun to eat more fish, so I also take a nightly DMSA capsule with selenium (and other synergistic factors) to further enhance my own ODP-based mercury detoxification program.

Recent research supports the increased benefits from using both EDTA and DMSA, possibly even exceeding certain DMPS effects, without the associated costs and risks. EDTA is only five-to-eighteen percent absorbed, yet even the non-absorbed portion can help save your life. It will increase fecal levels of toxic metals pulling out the metals we are ingesting and also lower the level of free radical reactions going on in the intestines, decreasing the levels of mutagen and carcinogens in feces, and thus reducing the potential for colon cancer, while also decreasing the potential for entero-hepatic re-uptake of toxic metals. The absorbed portion of oral EDTA seems to activate many useful functions, such as a weak heparin-like effect from a mucopolysaccharide synergy, and never fails to consistently lower lead levels.

There is no single chelator that is ideal to detox all of the different tissues in our body, as some need fat-soluble and some need water-soluble metal chelators, and some are more alkaline or acid, etc. Thus truly effective detoxification requires the use of newly developing combinations of highly effective detoxifying nutrients and or drugs. These may include many of the substances I consider to be potential ancillary nutrients in my ODP: taurine, lipoic acid, stabilized fiber, stabilized ascorbic acid, rutosid. Silybin, a new iron chelating agent, stabilizes the unstable molecule formed by ascorbate in the presence of iron (III). Centella Asiatica improves the effects of DMSA. Curcumin is an effective iron chelator. Thiol compounds work better when concurrently administered with thiamine. There is an ongoing need for magnesium supplementation. All these are useful nutritional therapies to synergistically enhance the benefits from any other chelation program.

Wobenzym

One example of an important nutritional chelator is an iron chelator from China called rutosid in the original German Wobenzym formula which is now being made in Arizona. This iron chelator prevents bruising after major trauma or surgery if taken in adequate quantities up to ten tablets q.i.d. away from food, and long enough for healing to occur. They give 50 of these at once in emergency rooms in Germany where the product originally was perfected. Now, finally, we are able to produce it here in Arizona in a specialized plant designed for the complex task of making a natural non-toxic product that in expensive controlled studies competes head to head with Celebrex®.

The iron chelation effect from Wobenzym is due to the rutosid content. This effect is vital for the antioxidant and other well-documented benefits of Wobenzym. In the body, iron chelation is primarily handled by transferrin and ferritin. Free iron is extremely toxic and therefore must be bound (chelated) at all times, or it accelerates free radical damage and lipid peroxidation. Since we cannot increase the levels of these natural chelators ferritin or transferrin which the body uses to sequester free iron overnight, I use my ODP. For acute trauma following surgery, I also incorporate nutritional chelators with extra iron-binding effects, like Wobenzym. Its special form of rutosid sequesters the iron released by the surgery or injury with an appropriately charged "companion" so that the released iron molecules from the injury or surgery are no longer free metals. Thus, I can help prevent the iron from catalyzing free radicals.

A High-Value Vitamin C

The world today seems to be in a useless "horsepower race" to claim the latest and greatest high Oxygen Radical Absorbance Capacity (ORAC) value antioxidant from the latest new multi-level company. Most of this is hype, and high ORAC values alone are not enough to let us live a long life on a toxic planet. Fortunately, most of us take vitamin C supplements, but we know that they are not always providing the antioxidant effects we desire, unless concurrently ingested with some metal-binding agents such as are present in Bio En'R-G'y C, my new vitamin C product. Vitamin C generally appears to do many vital things, such as supporting collagen synthesis, so it is always helpful.

However, the non-stabilized forms of vitamin C on the market today do not appear to offer significant reactive oxygen species (ROS) inhibition, and therefore it is not surprising that, to date, no vitamin C study has shown significant long-term protection against developing cancer.

I wanted my daily oral vitamin C supplement to provide maximum antioxidant activity. I had little confidence in the widely used ORAC testing unless it is done with more testing to document the actual inhibition of ROS in biological tissues. This is much more expensive testing, of course, but vital if we are to develop the advanced nutritional formula we need now if we are to finally enjoy the true benefits that the right formula of oral vitamin C can provide. I believe we now have developed that formula with Bio En'R-G'y C with G.M.SñRibose, etc., that can work optimally in our toxic bodies and still provide meaningful and provable daily antioxidant activity in all the tissues where vitamin C is so vital.

I believe that combining ODP, with its metal-binding effects, with the new forms of vitamin C and fiber, a formula I have helped develop, may change that. In any event, most patients who want to may now take 8 to 16 grams a day orally without suffering gastrointestinal (GI) upset, diarrhea, or bowel irritation, thus providing one more important tool in my ODP: a well-tolerated, well-absorbed, high-dose, oral ascorbic acid without side effects. This, taken in conjunction with the stabilized rice bran in Beyond Fiber, rounds out my total ODP program.

This actually is another aspect of metal-binding in medicine, since I have found that by combining the new form of oral vitamin C with certain other natural chelators, vitamin C can provide these remarkable antioxidant effects at very low concentrations in tissue. Using tests that are more sophisticated than simple ORAC values, we have been able to document highly significant inhibiting of ROS in a biological study using human neutrophils even at parts-per-billion levels. No other vitamin C preparation comes close to delivering these effects. The chelators can help further stabilize this special form of vitamin C, and that may explain the almost complete lack of GI irritation seen with this new form of vitamin C, even when ingesting doses of 20 gm a day, as Linus Pauling recommended. Some report taking this dosage along with large doses of ODP products.

Occasionally, some patients are even taking this form of vitamin C in drinks, like the Penta® water I recommend for detoxification, and some also use Bio EnRGy with 2-3 gm of oral Calcium EDTA. Some have reported gratifying improvement in cardiovascular function, even regaining the ability to exercise vigorously. We are just beginning to learn how to maximize pro-oxidant and antioxidant therapies with metal-binding and/or chelating agents and various nutrients.

Other Additions To the ODP

My research convinces me that there are only minimal risks when consuming low levels of garlic, malic acid (apple acid), EDTA, and DMSA. This was documented in the case of EDTA by the FDA studies before they allowed EDTA to be added to any food, as a preservative, where interestingly EDTA was found to also lower free radical damage of the foods, just as I believe it is doing in our patients who are on my ODP.

We have documented hundreds of studies regarding the benefits of lower levels of toxic metals like lead and mercury, and since the risks with ODP are minimal, you can see why after using the basic program on my body for over 20 years without fail, I now think it is safe enough to give it in this new improved form as ODP to anyone, even our pets and horses. (In the future, farm animals may routinely need to start receiving some forms of ODP in their food and water, as there is no question that lowering toxins reduces all causes of morbidity and mortality, which is a large problem with turkey and chicken growers.) Using ODP means that all of us with lower toxic metals can live longer before diseases like diabetes, arthritis, heart disease or cancer develop, the appearance of illness will be delayed, and the severity will be less by lowering toxins.

Safety & New Products

Since the components of my ODP include numerous ingredients with extensive documentation pointing to their safety, I am comfortable proposing the radical idea of life-long continued detoxification, as long as patients always take the best possible high-potency mineral replacement product concurrently. With so many studies documenting safe substances available to help detox from garlic and malic acid to ascorbic acid and stabilized rice bran and oral EDTA, etc. I am not enthusiastic about any new chelator of the month, although I do carefully evaluate each, as we always need better therapies. Most new chelators that I look into turn out to be overly hyped and poorly studied with new cure-all claims.

I review all new information about detoxification products that come out. I always want to simplify and lower price, and I am always open to looking for better answers. Unfortunately, when I look at some products whose proponents claim 100% absorption, I find that the data falls apart on closer analysis. I have nothing against rectal applications but most medicines administered rectally are not better absorbed. Contrary to claims, such application really only avoids first pass metabolism by the liver. Considering the need for long-term detoxification, such nightly applications would soon irritate the tissues. And by not taking the oral program I am not suggesting that patients miss some important opportunities to decrease free radicals in the intestine, which should somewhat lower colon cancer incidence. I prefer having some antioxidant metal-binding going on in my intestine all the time, if just to diminish enterohepatic reuptake of heavy metals.

I have spent over two million dollars over the past 20 years on my postgraduate studies, and Part One of this article lists discoveries and studies that I have found that will deliver the punch we need to help patients facing increasingly serious diseases at younger and younger ages whose only hope often is an extremely toxic, often unaffordable drug that might help them live three more months. I hope to empower all *Townsend Letter* readers to make use of my experience to visit my website and perhaps join the FACT discussion group. I hope to empower you to provide meaningful interventions for thousands of patients. You may not have a cure for their condition, but if you study this detoxification concept, there will be no patients to whom you cannot offer meaningful intervention. Although there is no guarantee about overcoming the primary diagnosis, realistic detoxification can help when no other approach is available.

It seems that some see an effective oral detoxification program such as my ODP as a threat rather than a way to help thousands of additional patients. I do not find that there is a magic wand available anywhere. However, I challenge anyone to review and argue against the documentation supporting what I am saying here. You can view much of it conveniently for no charge on my website anytime. A group of chelating doctors wanted me to debate them about the value of oral chelation over IV chelation. They all saw IV as essential to the economic well-being of their practices, so the moderator said it would be unfair for me to pass out anything that had all the references supporting my case.

My ODP is more accepting of patient needs. For example, type in the word Coumadin® on my website to review my position and see how I let patients decide for themselves whether to combine my oral programs (with things like Boluoke added to the oral chelation where warranted) or to replace Coumadin® entirely. Coumadin® is one of the most dangerous drugs prescribed, and responsible prescribers today should do genetic testing to determine the rate of metabolism of Coumadin® to help avoid the all-too-frequent bleeding episodes that kill patients and put so many in the hospital for little long-term benefit. I find its effects to be weak compared to those of the ODP.

I have never encountered a bleeding episode at any time with the safe, gentle, heparin-like activity produced by EDTA, which requires the presence of the correct form of mucopolysaccharide. Note: Heparin has a strong negative charge, and there are other substances with that charge. EDTA helps those other substances work orally. I also support other nutrients to increase this heparin-like effect, and the literature supports this idea of oral heparin. Other additions, like Wobenzym with its papain and bromelain components will also enhance oral heparin absorption, while Wobenzym's overall anti-inflammatory effect helps to lower the viscosity that inflammation increases.

Once you understand that substantially increasing your patient's life span generally cannot be accomplished with any intervention that is followed for only a few weeks or even months, then you may decide to use some substances for many years. And when you do so, it would be prudent to have those substances already proven safe by years of documented use. There are nearly 50 years of reported experience around the substances I am discussing here like EDTA, garlic, malic acid, ascorbic acid, fiber, etc.

We know that DMSA is normally found in the body; it too is quite safe when used appropriately. Malic acid (apple acid) is amazingly useful for multipurpose detoxifying, almost working on aluminum as well as desferoxamine. This leaves us with many safe, synergistic, metal-binding substances like garlic, vitamin C, and fiber, all of which I believe should be part of any long-term successful ODP. I am convinced such a program will add years to your lives and life to those years.

I first worked with Dr. Lester Morrison over 20 years ago. We came out with earlier versions of the basic ODP program, based on his three textbooks and his two documented studies showing a 91% reduction in fatal heart attacks in patients on his Institute Formula. We later determined EDTA dramatically enhanced the formula's effects, so that the product could be taken in the three capsules of Essential Daily Defense we now use twice daily as part of the basic nine-tablet package of pills. The EDTA permitted the desired effects to be achieved with a far lower dose and still provide the desired anti-clotting protection. I routinely encourage symptomatic patients to initially concurrently take 30 or more of the older three-hour IV chelation or the new painless calcium EDTA, the new short chelation sweeping the world today.

I have also helped to develop EDTA-containing gum, called EZ Defense, which I feel at least minimizes some of the toxic exposure from amalgam fillings if used immediately after each meal, since chewing releases mercury from amalgam.   This gum approach is an addition to the life-long oral chelation program that I know will keep my patient alive and healthy even with a mouthful of amalgam fillings. I am confident that even with ten amalgam fillings, my patients on such a program will outlive those who spend the money to remove their dental mercury. This is because those patients spend so much time and money on just dealing with mercury removal, which is only one source of their total body burden, they cannot conceive that they still must spend still more money every month and stay on a lifetime ODP program. I believe this is essential if we are to help them achieve their maximum intended useful lifespan enjoying anything like the optimal health I have been fortunate enough to enjoy since learning all this years ago.

If your patient can remove their amalgam fillings and stay on the totally ODP program for life, well and good. However, I still prefer to postpone the dental work until my patients have begun to show real signs of recovery. This is because no matter how careful the dentist is, there is always a strong likelihood of a short-term significantly increased mercury exposure for a time with any amalgam removal.

If due to finances I have to recommend an even simpler, less comprehensive basic program for detoxification I use just stabilized vitamin C, EDTA and the special stabilized rice bran in combination with a special source of inulin as my vital FIBER contribution to detoxification everyday of life, as well as for the probiotic effects. Those three items comprise an affordable program that can dramatically reduce all causes of morbidity and mortality. This may seem expensive, but we all know the costs of a single emergency visit for chest pain or one hospitalization. It is a sad fact that over 50% of the money spent on health care for the average person is spent in the final year of life. That money does very little to change the final outcome. I recommend spending some money every month now for my ODP program to significantly improve the quality and quantity of life.

Dealing with Causes of Toxicity

I never recommend any form of ODP for long-term use without concurrent aggressive nutritional supplementation. As mentioned above, many people experience the effects of mercury exposure from dental amalgam fillings. Today's levels of environmental toxicity also increase the need for most nutrients. Thus the Recommended Daily Allowances (RDA) have no real applicability when we design programs to treat toxic people. And who today is not toxic? The National Health and Nutrition Examination Survey (NHANES) study, funded by the National Institutes of Health (NIH) corroborates what the Environmental Working Group (EWG) reported when they found that everyone from all walks of life have 40-plus neurotoxins in the blood at all times.

The EWG studies were done at Mt. Sinai School of Medicine. The study measured up to 240 chemicals per patient. And in *Plague Time*, author Paul Ewald documents that virtually everyone today has some CMV, Chlamydia, herpes, SV40 or even cell wall infections. Clearly, we all possess numerous neurotoxins and carcinogens, and no one tested is free of significant numbers of such toxins, even if you live an all-organic life, since you are still living on our toxic planet.

Birds in remote mountain areas of the United States have been found to have frighteningly high levels of mercury. Researchers have proven that mercury and other heavy metals in these birds at high elevations are proven to be coming from coal-burning power plants from as far away as China. In fact, radio isotope analysis of the mercury proves we too are consuming mercury coming from the burning of coal in far off China. China and India are slated to bring online hundreds of new coal burning power plants over the next few years. There is a report that as little as one new coal burning plant in Texas seemed to increase the incidence of autism there by 17%. These new plants will dump tons of mercury into the environment.

This information makes me considerably less aggressive about removing just one source of the pollution. I do not focus excessively on just one source of toxicity, whether it be vaccines or fillings or fish. Our genetics, environment, and diet are the interplay that largely determines the outcome from our ongoing continuous heavy metal exposures, which are all cumulative.

Getting the Lead Out

Of course, good medical practice requires identifying specific extra sources of exposure. This can be amazing, and I have saved lives by being a Sherlock Holmes. Why not devise a program that helps to deal with all the heavy metals in my patients and never stops working, one that can be most likely implemented for less cost than might be spent dealing with just the dental contribution to the overall body burden of toxic heavy metals?

I have identified and removed major sources of toxicity in my years of following up on abnormal blood, urine, and hair heavy metal testing as director at one time of MINERALAB, then the largest trace element testing lab in the world, subsequently acquired by Doctor's Data. I have written books that identify all the possible contributors that can aggravate the overall toxicity that I am focusing on in this article. These toxins include certain eating utensils to lead paint in homes, even lead linings in bathtubs and, of course, lead paints and lead in drinking water.

Again, we need to learn to look at the total body burden of toxins and not simply focus on just one problem, such as the obvious mercury exposure in vaccines, dental amalgams, or particular fish. Lead is always there and easy-to-treat. For any heavy metal exposure, always try to deal with the lead too, as it makes the other exposures worse, and treatment is both easy and cost-effective. This approach is essential if we are to provide optimal benefits to patients, whether you are dealing with a depressed mercury-exposed dentist, who may also have associated cardiovascular disease, or a hyperactive child.

Anytime my ODP does NOT find significantly improved levels on toxic metal retesting in any tissue three to four months after starting, my experience has been that we have a persistent source of heavy metal that must be identified and removed. Anyone being treated for mercury should also be treated for lead, since lead makes mercury up to 100 times more toxic. That is why my ODP uses many metal-binding agents, including EDTA, DMSA, selenium, garlic, etc.

Remember, all heavy metals drag down the immunity, so there, almost routinely, will be an increased total body burden of pathogens that may need concurrent treatment with something, perhaps, oxidative therapies, or antibiotics, etc. which I will be helping teach at the oxidative workshops offered by ACAM.

Autism and Metal Toxicity

I have reviewed extensive documentation, from Doctor's Data, involving over 10,000 data points from our autism protocol research. The children on that program always saw substantial improvement, even after all prior attempts had failed completely (or even made the child worse), no matter the age. Whether the patient is 5 years old or 20, the potential for favorable response to the program does not diminish, although, admittedly, the protocol for autism requires more detail than I am covering in this article. That protocol requires great attention to all details, as covered on my DVDs and in the books on autism that I have co-authored (please see www.gordonresearch.com).

The program that I have helped teach, and have written about extensively, has convinced me that there are genetic issues involving methylation in all autistic children. I find those same genetic issues also contribute to many other chronic, neurodegenerative diseases, such as Alzheimer's disease, multiple sclerosis, ALS, etc. These mutations impair the body's ability to excrete heavy metals and control viral infections. This helps set the stage for lowered immunity, which then permits the infections we all carry to take off. Effective methylation is essential for effective detoxification as well as for infection control throughout life. A total program is necessary, taking a few years to gradually but continuously achieve success.

The autistic children studied generally have also been shown to have live virus. Some of their viral load seems to be the same as the virus injected with their MMR vaccinations. These vaccinations for a time were being given with thimerosal- (an organomercurial; i.e., mercury). Of course no one is doing routine genetic testing yet on all newborns, so no one knew that these children were genetically "at risk." The environmental degradation that pollutes our environment with increasing mercury simply sets the stage for more children to be unable to handle the stress of vaccines. Although since much of the thimerosal has now been removed from those vaccines, there seems to be some decrease in the overall incidence of autism. However, environmental toxicity just increases. For instance, we have the new coal-burning power plants in India and China that may fill that "void" and bring mercury levels back up to that time when all vaccines contained mercury.

The vaccines clearly have often been reported by parents to be the straw that pushes the child over the brink. Soon after the vaccines, these children change; they lose speech. Many different infections are complicating the diagnosis and treatment of heavy metal poisoning; there are numerous infections documented to hold heavy metals. Study this by learning that Coxackie infections can hold 70 times too much cadmium in the infected tissues. This is a vital point about detoxification requiring concurrent treatment of the pathogen load if we hope to get at the critical heavy metals that are impairing function such as loss of speech in a child. These infections fool doctors into believing there are no more heavy metals to treat, leaving patients treated incompletely.

It is shocking but true that often the toughest children we have treated would have previously shown only very little or no mercury excretion after IV DMPS, with the well-meaning doctors who treated them. Sometimes doctors gave up and mistakenly informed the parents that there was no mercury in their autistic child. They conclude erroneously that any heavy metal detoxification with chelation would not help. I hope this article helps gets the right information out to everyone.

That information was totally wrong. The total detoxification program we developed always increases excretion of heavy metals, and when this begins, we see substantial clinical improvement follow. We only need to use gentle oral EDTA, malic acid and/or garlic, MSM, lipoic acid, etc. (i.e., ODP) as our primary oral treatment, and over time, we almost invariably start to find mercury released, or tin or antimony or cadmium or aluminum or lead. These metals were not coming up with previous use of IV chelators because of genetics and infection problems. There is always increased excretion of toxic metals seen with the correct program, sometimes more in feces than in urine.

There is, however, no rhyme or reason regarding what comes first. Sometimes these metals would almost be off the chart in some children when we used fecal and/or urine testing with Doctor's Data, even though the poor results with standard IV provocation caused the family and doctor to think that there was no mercury or other toxic metal present. Sometimes tin is the metal excreted for three months, then antimony for three months, then lead, and finally, a year later, mercury or aluminum.

These metals will not come out, even with intravenous application of DMPS, until a total program is developed and followed wherein the body's overall health is raised sufficiently to permit overcoming these infections. That, in addition, with immune supporting and RNA-based therapies permits the patient's body to overcome this total body burden of infection. When the viral load finally starts to leave the body, we often find immediately thereafter significant spikes in the excretion of the heavy metals, which many times had not been chelatable before that anti-pathogen treatment began to work, even with aggressive intravenous application of chelating agents in these children.

Infections may promote local tissue increases in metallothionein, which can be a very potent chelator, and may have a higher stability constant, thus sequestering the metal in the infected tissue more tightly than the concentration of chelating agent in the affected tissue, even when the EDTA and/or DMSA or DMPS or other chelators were being administered intravenously. (I seldom use DMPS as I do not like the benefit-to-risk ratio.)

We can turn around even the toughest cases, given time and adequate family support. Remember, there is no cure for these infections that are holding the metals, so we have to help the child get well enough to overcome the infections. This can be even more difficult when there is also be a genetic component, such as the COMT gene. From birth, these patients are markedly impaired in their ability to excrete heavy metals. This means we have to use our comprehensive protocol, which concurrently treats all aspects of the problem; ideally, this needs to be personalized, based on genetic test results.

Also, always, we remove all suspect foods from our patients' diets; these may include all gluten foods—not just wheat, dairy, and corn—and any other foods where testing or history makes them suspect. I also have these patients eliminate all soft drinks, particularly those with high fructose corn syrup. In addition, we have to clean up their total environment, including chemicals stored in the home. We also must treat the total body burden of pathogens, and many will be excited to learn more about how to do this with oxidative therapies at ACAM. This is particularly vital for most chronic degenerative diseases, including heart disease, multiple sclerosis to Parkinson's, etc., not just autism.

I also have been impressed with Alinia® and Daxon as drug treatments that deal with frequently under-diagnosed serious parasite issues. These are commonly missed with standard stool testing. This parasite problem is almost another subspecialty and needs motivated and trained specialists to diagnosis and treat. I sometimes treat empirically, as we do for horses and dogs, as I am convinced that far too many of the parasites today are not amenable to simple herbal therapies. I recommend learning about drugs like Alinia or Daxon, as it's known in Mexico, where the drug is less expensive.

Summary

It is not the purpose of this article to duplicate the over 60 hours of teaching we have done in the past three years at our semi-annual conferences, all of which are on DVDs. I only want to cover a few highlights that might stimulate a broader interest on the part of all *Townsend Letter* readers to learn that, whatever your practice, you probably have been given misinformation regarding metal binding, bio-inorganic chemistry, and chelation, and that misinformation is most likely seriously impairing your ability to serve your patients optimally.

Our lifetime accumulations of heavy metals begin at conception, and I advocate detoxing prospective parents. This means we need to start ODP as early as possible, at preconception, and continue though gestation. This means pregnant patients must always also be on their mandatory concurrent aggressive oral supplementation program. You may also check for malabsorption so that no potential zinc deficiency develops. There can be legitimate criticism regarding use of ODP during pregnancy, particularly if you include EDTA. EDTA was reported in rodents to induce mutagenesis, but the evidence showed that adequate zinc replacement eliminated that problem. My website covers informed consent issues for problems like Coumadin® replacement to nutritionally based practices. I am convinced that most chronic health conditions in any human or animal will respond better to the chosen treatment plan for their condition if concurrent use of my ODP were employed.

In conclusion, as I summarize this article, I also offer these key points to remember (in no particular order):

IV Chelation therapy can significantly improve cardiovascular status without necessarily reversing atherosclerosis, which in fact occasionally worsens.

Optimal heavy metal detoxification also may need to concurrently lower the total body burden of pathogens. The total body burden of pathogens can be treated with oxidative therapies.

Selenium is an extremely low-cost strategy that appropriately used may significantly help deal with many mercury issues.

The Environmental Protection Agency's journal, *Environmental Health Perspectives*, publishes vital documentation regarding the dangers of lead, mercury, cadmium, tin, antimony, uranium, aluminum, etc.

The American Board of Clinical Metal Toxicology, under Robert Nash, MD, attempts to help set standards in the area of clinical metal toxicology.

Negative provoked urine tests using IV chelating agent(s) do not rule out the significant probability that a patient still has a significantly increased body burden of heavy metals, which may be revealed with X-ray fluorescence, which can determine bone lead levels. Bone lead is not innocuous and is in equilibrium with tissues throughout the body, and therefore elevated bone lead is associated with earlier development of cataracts. This corroborates the obvious fact that lead is then not just in bone but in kidney, spleen, liver, heart and brain, as well as the eye.

Ideal metal-binding agents should be those that are quite safe for long-term use. Average bone turn-over for adults is fifteen years; therefore, a realistic program for heavy metal detoxification should always be planned for a minimum of fifteen years.

The ideal agents that we find have unique synergy today include DMSA, EDTA, malic acid, garlic, fiber, selenium, penicillamine, desferoxamine, vitamin C, rutosid, lipoic acid, taurine, silybin. These are some nutrients that are ancillary to enhancing the effectiveness of oral chelators such as DMSA.

The growing fetus is used by the mother's body as a toxic dump site for the mercury, and toxic metals all bioaccumulate in the growing fetus, leading to over 600,000 children born with elevated mercury levels at birth.

A hair test showing low levels of mercury may mean nothing as it simply may be a patient with a genetic issue impairing the excretion of heavy metals; such a patient may need ODP much more than some patients with higher levels of hair mercury.

Rapidly increasing utilization of coal-burning electric power plants in

China and other places around the world is dramatically increasing the level of pollution and degrading our environment.

Metal-binding agents/chelating agents have many vital functions in the body. Antioxidants, including ascorbic acid, under certain conditions, can become pro-oxidant. There is some research showing the binding of transition metal by metal-binding agents can help avoid that pro-oxidant status.

EDTA orally administered with heparin-like compounds (mucopoly-saccharide) may be a safe alternative to Coumadin®, Plavix®, or even aspirin, decreasing clots and lowering blood viscosity for fully informed and consenting patients.

My website, www.Gordonresearch.com/townsend, has approximately ten thousand pages of information searchable by using the 'Search,' so a search on mercury will receive over 181 interesting articles that I have managed to accumulate on that narrowed topic.

I find it is not essential to select a treatment that crosses the blood brain barrier to get excellent results in treating chronic neurotoxicity. The simple laws of diffusion support the fact that if you continue slowly to always be pulling more mercury and other toxins out of the body than is coming in, over time, you will have lower and lower levels in plasma, serum, extra cellular fluids, brain tissue, etc. We lose ten billion cells everyday.

We all need to learn more about bio-inorganic chemistry, which is another word for metal-binding in medicine. There are textbooks with these exact titles. In fact, when I was first researching chelation, the very first book I got was from Lippincott and was entitled *Metal Binding in Medicine*. It explained how the concept of chelation had virtually leapt from the laboratory into clinical medicine. These were the published proceedings of a conference held in 1959, put on by Dr. Seven. That book changed my life, and I hope I motivate some reader to pick up this subject matter, as pollution will not go away and we need better and better answers.

Pathologic calcification of vascular tissues can be effectively diagnosed and treated and even reversed with a program that I have written extensively about the includes vitamin K-2, along with aggressive vitamin C supplementation along with Pueraria Mirificia, strontium, and boron etc. This program also seems to routinely prevent and even reverse osteoporosis without using the drugs being prescribed, which have very substantial dangerous side effects.

Vitamin K2 research particularly menaquinone-7 clearly has been documented with extensive studies at the University of Maastricht in Holland to be an important part of the answer to dealing with calcification of vascular tissues.

Everyone adequately tested today will be found positive for some forms of Chlamydia, CMV, herpes, SV40, and possibly Lyme. Appropriately administered oxidative therapies will lower the total body burden of pathogens.

EDTA is only 5-18% absorbed, yet even the non-absorbed portion can help save your life. It will increase fecal levels of toxic metals, pulling out the metals we are ingesting. EDTA will also lower the level of free-radical reactions going on in the intestines, decreasing the levels of mutagen and carcinogens in feces, and thus reducing the potential for colon cancer, while also decreasing the potential for entero-hepatic re-uptake of toxic metals. The absorbed portion oral EDTA seems to activate many useful functions, such as a weak heparin-like effect from a mucopolysaccharide synergy, and never fails to consistently lower lead levels.

Menopausal women frequently become hypertensive. New research recognizes a relationship between bone loss and increasing release of lead from those bones causing low-level lead toxicity. This may lead to increased blood pressure as well as adversely affecting all aspects of the immune system. This suggests that long-term lowering of bone lead stores can have many hidden benefits. We now have an epidemic of disabled children, including those affected by autism, and evidence of dramatically increasing levels of heavy metals in all living organisms everywhere on earth. We now have extensive documentation regarding the adverse effects of these heavy metals on our lifespan, on all causes of morbidity and mortality, and on our IQ and worker productivity, etc.

My work in the field of autism confirms that beyond question there are many infections in these children. These infections are responsible for holding onto toxic metals, including antimony, tin, uranium, aluminum, lead, mercury, cadmium.

As the world becomes more toxic, even farmers will have to look into their cost benefit ratio in considering life time detoxification of their herds. This may lead to preventatively treating hogs, chickens, cattle and work animals. My work with performance animals has indicated that those who were treated with the Beyond Fiber, the Beyond C and the Essential Daily Defense products that I formulated for Longevity Plus were able to go from average performing, non-Blue Ribbon winning average horses to Grand Prix champions.

We need to offer some effective long-term answer to the problems I've detailed in this article, and my ODP provides a long-term solution. It may be a little late to stop the polluters, so we all need the ODP to enhance excretions of these toxins. Please feel free to challenge these ideas. They represent an overview from my 35 years of involvement in chelation therapy, during which time, I have been a co-founder 35 years ago of what is now called ACAM and a co-founder of the American Board of Chelation Therapy, which has now become the American Board of Clinical Metal Toxicology, an organization I serve as advisor.

I hope this information proves valuable to you in your own health, and in helping to improve the health of your patients.

GLOSSARY

advanced glycation end-products (AGEs): Sticky unions of sugar and protein that are created in the body when excess circulating sugar molecules bind to proteins and combine with them, creating cross-linked proteins that gum up the body's vital enzymes and increase free-radical damage. AGEs have been linked to numerous diseases, and are known to accelerate aging in general. Age spots on the skin and cataracts in the lens of the eye are examples of AGE formation.

angina pectoris: Acute recurring chest pain or discomfort resulting from a decreased blood supply to the heart muscle (known as myocardial ischemia). Angina is a common symptom of coronary heart disease, and it occurs when the heart's need for oxygen increases beyond the level of oxygen that is available from the blood nourishing the heart.

agonist: A substance that binds to a receptor on a cell and triggers an action or a response by the cell, often mimicking the action of a naturally occurring substance. An agonist is the opposite of an antagonist, which binds to a cell and blocks an action.

amino acids: Simple organic compounds containing nitrogen which are the building blocks of proteins.

arteriosclerosis: A disease of the blood vessels caused by plaque deposits and characterized by a narrowing and a hardening of the arteries, as well as by a loss of elasticity, which causes a decrease in blood flow and increases the risk of a heart attack or stroke. (In Greek "arterio" means "artery" and "sclerosis" means "hardening".)

atherosclerosis: A form of arteriosclerosis (see: **arteriosclerosis**) specifically due to an accumulation of atheromatous plaque—anatomic lesions that result from an accumulation of inflammatory cells, fats and other lipids, and connective tissue within the walls of arteries. (In Greek "athero" means "porridge" and "sclerosis" means "hardening".)

antioxidant: A chemical that prevents the oxidative degradation of other chemicals and helps to neutralize free radicals in the body.

ATP (adenosine triphosphate): A nucleotide, produced by the mitochondria inside cells, that is responsible for the chemical energy that drives otherwise uphill biochemical reactions in the body.

axons: A thin branch that transmits electrical impulses away from neurons (brain cells) to other neurons, muscles, or glands.

bioflavonoids: Bioflavonoids are a class of water-soluble plant pigments that are naturally found in fruits and vegetables. Although they are not considered essential, they are reported to have numerous health benefits, as anti-inflammatory, antihistaminic, and anti-viral agents.

biosphere: The outermost part of the Earth's crust—which contains the oceans, continents and atmosphere—in which all biological processes occur. The biosphere is a self-organizing system, whereby the waste from some of the organisms (plants) serve as the nutrients for other organisms (animals) and vice versa.

Biosphere 2: The largest artificial, self-sustaining ecosystem ever built. A completely sealed, glass-enclosed 3.15 acre environment, built in the Oracle, Arizona desert. Biosphere 2 is composed of miniature replicas of all the earth's environments, and it houses 3,800 species of plants and animals, designed to function together as a single system.

biospherian: A subject in the original Biosphere 2 (See: Biosphere 2) experiments. One of the people who lived and worked for a set period of time—the longest time being two years—inside the artificial, self-sustaining ecosystem.

C-reactive protein (CRP): An acute phase protein produced by the liver that increases during systemic inflammation. Testing CRP levels in the blood may be useful as way to assess cardiovascular disease risk, as elevated CRP levels are correlated with a higher incidence of coronary artery disease.

chelation: A natural chemical process that goes on continually in our bodies, in which a metal or mineral becomes bonded to another substance.

chelation therapy: A form of oral or intravenous therapy that employs a chemical agent that binds readily with heavy metals so as to help remove them from the body.

chemokine: A type of peptide which causes specific immune cells to move toward a chemical stimulus.

cross-linking: The process of chemically joining two or more molecules by a covalent bond; i.e., when electrons are shared between atoms. This sometimes results in the formation of abnormal chemical bonds between adjacent protein strands, which deforms them and impairs their function in the body.

dendrites: Tiny tree-like branchings at the electrical impulse-receiving end of a neuron (brain cell).

dioxins: A general term that describes a group of hundreds of highly toxic chemicals that are present in our biosphere. It is formed as an unintentional byproduct of many industrial processes involving chlorine, such as waste incineration and pesticide manufacturing.

DNA: Deoxyribonucleic acid—the long complex macromolecule, consisting of two interconnected helical strands, that resides in the nucleus of every living cell and encodes the genetic instructions for building each organism.

double-blind: A type of scientific or clinical study in which neither the subject nor the experimenter know if the subject is receiving an experimental treatment or a placebo. This controls for the effects of expectation and belief.

ejection fraction: The amount of blood pumped out of a ventricle with each heart beat, which is used as a measurement of the heart's efficiency. The ejection fraction is calculated by the amount of blood pumped by the heart divided by the amount of blood the ventricle contains.

endogenous: Found naturally within the body; produced within an organism. The opposite of exogenous.

enterohepatic reuptake: When the bile acids that are produced by the liver, and secreted into the small intestine in order to help the body digest fats and transport many waste products and toxins, is absorbed back into the blood stream in the lower part of the small intestine. It is because of this process that the body has such difficulty removing certain toxins and heavy metals from the body.

endothelium: A layer of thin specialized cells that line the interior surface of blood vessels throughout the entire circulatory system, from the heart to the smallest capillary.

essential nutrient: Components of food that are required for normal body functioning which can not be synthesized by the body. Essential nutrients include vitamins, minerals, essential fatty acids, and essential amino acids.

estrogen: A group of three steroid compounds (estradiol, estriol and estrone) that functions as the primary female sex hormone. Estrogen promotes the development of female secondary sex characteristics, such as breasts, and is involved in regulating the menstrual cycle.

evolutionary epidemiology: An emerging scientific field that integrates Darwinian evolutionary theory with the study of the causes, distribution, and control of disease in populations.

exogenous: Derived or developed outside of the body or organism. The opposite of endogenous.

excitatory neurotransmitter: A type of neurotransmitter—such as dopamine—that excites, speeds up, or accelerates neural processes. The opposite of an inhibitory neurotransmitter, which slows down neural processes.

free radical: Highly reactive atoms or molecules with unpaired electrons. Free radicals can cause substantial oxidative damage to the body and are thought to be one of the primary causes of aging. Because free radicals are necessary for normal metabolism, the body uses antioxidants to minimize free radical-induced damage.

genome: The complete set of genetic material or genes for a single organism.

genomic testing: Tests which scan an individual's DNA for gene variants, acquired mutations, and measure gene expression. Genomic testing can be helpful in predicting an individual's predisposition towards many dangerous genetic diseases. This allows people to take preventive measures, and for physicians to modify gene expression through precise, targeted, individualized interventions.

germ-line cells: The body's sex cells (sperm and ovum), whose function is to propagate the individual's DNA through sexual reproduction.

glycation: A chemical reaction between proteins and sugars, which results in toxic products that are thought to be one of the primary causes of aging.

HDL: High-density lipoprotein, the "good" cholesterol, which removes cholesterol from the arteries before it has a chance to oxidize, and reduces the inflammatory process. Higher HDL levels are correlated with a lower incidence of cardiovascular disease.

homocysteine: Toxic metabolic byproducts formed by eating methionine, an amino acid found in animal protein foods like poultry and red meat. Elevated homocysteine levels are associated with a greater risk of cardiovascular disease.

hormone: A chemical messenger produced in one part of the body that is carried through the bloodstream to other parts of the body, where it invokes a specific response. These responses vary widely, but they can include stimulating new cell growth, regulating metabolism, or preparing the body for a new phase of life, such as puberty or menopause. They may also stimulate a behavioral response, such as fleeing, fighting, or mating.

LDL: Low-density lipoprotein, the "bad" cholesterol. The oxidation of LDL in the arteries is the first step toward vulnerable plaque formation, which leads to cardiovascular disease.

inhibitory neurotransmitter: A type of neurotransmitter—such as serotonin—that inhibits or slows down neural processes. The opposite of an excitatory neurotransmitter, which accelerates neural processes.

metastatic calcium: Calcium that has been deposited into living tissue. This form of calcium causes the blood vessels to harden and leads to arteriosclerosis.

mitochondria: Structures within cells that produce energy by respiratory metabolism. Mitochondria have their own DNA and are thought to be bacteria that were captured by animal cells in the course of evolution.

MRI (Magnetic Resonance Imaging) Scan: A diagnostic technique that detects structures by their different content of atoms with certain resonances to induced magnetic fields and produces very detailed, two or three-dimensional, cross-sectional images of organs inside the body. It is especially useful for viewing soft tissue and doesn't use X-rays or any dangerous form of radiation.

myocardial infarction: A disease state that occurs when the blood supply to a part of the heart muscle is interrupted, commonly known as a heart attack. The resulting oxygen shortage (or ischemia) causes damage and potential death of heart tissue.

nanotechnology: Atomic engineering—the ability to devise self-replicating machines, robots, and computers on a molecular level.

nanobots: Self-replicating, molecule-sized robots.

neuropeptide: Peptides that are found in the brain and nervous system. (See: **peptides**)

neurotransmitter: Chemicals that transmit and modulate electrical signals between neurons (brain cells) and other cells.

nitric oxide: A highly reactive, gaseous chemical compound—composed of nitrogen and oxygen—that plays an important role in the body as a signaling molecule. Nitric oxide helps to control the circulation of the blood and regulate activities of the brain, lungs, liver, kidneys, stomach, genitals, and other organs.

paradigm: A model for explaining a set of data; a belief system.

paradigm shift: A change in the perception of information that often leads to a revolution in science.

PCBs: (Polychlorinated biphenyls): An unnatural mixture of up to 209 different highly toxic chlorinated compounds that were used as coolants and lubricants in electrical equipment. Because of evidence that they accumulate in the environment and can cause harmful health effects, in 1977 the manufacture of PCBs was halted in the U.S.—although they are still being released from hazardous waste sites. PCBs do not break down easily and remain in the environment for many years.

peptides: Strings consisting of two or more amino acids linked end to end. Peptides are used as chemical messengers that communicate information between systems in the body.

PET (Positron Emission Tomography) Scan: A powerful computer-generated, imaging technique that allows physicians and researchers to see a region of the body's metabolic activity in action. PET scans rely upon the detection of gamma rays, which are emitted from tissues after the administration of radioactive glucose—which circulates throughout the body, and is more readily metabolized in those cells that are more active.

phytochemical: A naturally-occurring, plant-derived chemical substance with biological activity—such as chlorophyll, beta-carotene, or lycopene. Many phytochemicals—which give plants their color, flavor, smell, and texture—are known to improve health and prevent disease.

phytoestrogens: Estrogen-like substances found in plants, especially soy. Some isoflavones (a type of phytochemical) are classified as phytoestrogens because their chemical structure is similar to human estrogen, and they act as weak estrogens in the body. Phytoestrogens are associated with a lowered risk of many diseases, including heart disease, osteoporosis and breast cancer.

placebo: An inactive substance, such as a sugar pill, which is tested blindly against an active substance to compensate for a possible effect created through the power of belief.

placebo effect: A measurable effect created by expectation and the power of belief.

RNA (Ribonucleic acid): A single-stranded nucleic acid (similar in structure to the double-stranded nucleic acid DNA) found inside of cells—in the nucleus and the cytoplasm—that plays an important information-transfering role in protein synthesis and other chemical activities of the cell.

silent inflammation: Inflammation is a characteristic reaction of tissues to injury or disease that is marked by swelling, redness, heat, and usually pain. However, there is a common form of inflammation known as 'silent inflammation' that is painless but extremely dangerous. Silent inflammation, which is often linked to diet, has been correlated with a higher incidence of cardiovascular disease, neurodegenerative disorders, cancer, and other illnesses.

standard deviation: A statistic that tells you how closely all of the various examples in a set of data are clustered around the average of that data. When the examples are tightly bunched together the standard deviation is small and when the examples are spread apart then the standard deviation is large. Smaller standard deviations imply less variation between subjects in scientific experiments, and larger standard deviations imply more variation.

testosterone: A steroid hormone from the androgen group that functions as the principal male sex hormone. Testosterone promotes the development of male secondary sex characteristics, such as facial hair, and is involved in regulating sperm production.

tocopherols: A component of vitamin E, a fat-soluble vitamin, which is composed of four tocopherols and four tocotrienols. The four tocopherols and the four tocotrienols are known as isomers because they are chemically similar but arranged differently. Each tocopherol has an alpha, beta, gamma, and delta form, and each form has its own biological activity.

tocotrienols: A component of vitamin E, a fat-soluble vitamin, which is composed of four tocotrienols and four tocopherols. The four tocotrienols and four tocopherols are known as isomers because they are chemically similar but arranged differently. Each tocotrienol has an alpha, beta, gamma, and delta form, and each form has its own biological activity.

vitamin: An organic compound that is essential for normal metabolism, which can not be synthesized by the body and must be supplied through the diet.

NOTES & REFERENCES

Introduction

1. Casdorph H.R. "EDTA chelation therapy, efficacy in arteriosclerotic heart disease." *J Holistic Medicine*, 1981; 3(1): 53.

2. Blumer W. and Cranton E.M. "Ninety percent reduction in cancer mortality after chelation therapy with EDTA." *J Adv Med*, 1989; 2: 183.

3. Hancke C. and Flythe K. "Benefits of EDTA Chelation Therapy on Arteriosclerosis: A Retrospective Study of 470 Patients." *Journal of Advancement in Medicine*, 1993; 6(3): 161.

4. Chappell L. T. and Stahl J.P. "The Correlation between EDTA Chelation Therapy and Improvement in Cardiovascular Function: A Meta-Analysis," *A Textbook on EDTA Chelation Therapy* (Second Edition), edited by Elmer M. Cranton, Hampton Roads Publishing, Virginia, 2001, 294-316.

5. Chappell L. T., Stahl J.P., and Evans R. "EDTA Chelation Treatment for Vascular Disease: A Meta-Analysis Using Unpublished Data," *A Textbook on EDTA Chelation Therapy* (Second Edition), edited by Elmer M. Cranton, Hampton Roads Publishing, Virginia, 2001, 317-328.

6. Cranton E.M. "Introduction to the Second Edition," *A Textbook on EDTA Chelation Therapy* (Second Edition), edited by Elmer M. Cranton, Hampton Roads Publishing, Virginia, 2001, xxi-xxxviii.

7. Rudolph C.J., Samuels R.T., McDonagh E.W. "Visual field evidence of macular degeneration reversal using a combination of EDTA chelation and multiple vitamin and trace mineral therapy." *Journal of Advancement in Medicine*, Winter, 1994; 7(4).

8. Hancke C., *ibid*.

9. Rudolph C.J., McDonagh E.W., and Wussow D. G. "The Effect of Intravenous Disodium Ethylenediaminetetraacetic Acid (EDTA) upon Bone Density Levels." *Journal of Advancement in Medicine*, 1988; 1(2): 79-85.

10. Gmerek D.E., et al. "Effect of inorganic lead on rat brain mitochondrial respiration and energy production." *J Neurochem*. 1981 Mar; 36(3): 1109-13.

11. Deucher G.P. "EDTA chelation therapy: an antioxidant strategy." *Journal of Advancement in Medicine*, 1988; 1(4): 182-190.

12. Casdorph H.R. "EDTA chelation therapy II, efficacy in brain disorders." *J Holistic Medicine*, 1981; 3(2): 101.

13. Clarke N.E., Clarke C.N., and Mosher R.E. "The "in vivo" dissolution of metastatic calcium: an approach to atherosclerosis." *Am J Med Sci*, 1955; 220: 142-149.

14. Clarke N.E., Clarke C.N., and Mosher R.E. "Treatment of Angina Pectoris With Disodium Ethylene Diamine Tetraacetic Acid." *American Journal of the Medical Sciences*, Dec., 1956; 232: 654-666.

15. Clarke, Sr., N.E., Clarke, Jr., N.E., and Mosher R.E. "Treatment of occlusive vascular disease with disodium ethylenediamine tetraacetic acid (EDTA)." *American Journal of Medical Science*, 1960; 239:732-44.

16. Chappell T.L. and Stahl J.P. "The correlation between EDTA chelation therapy and improvement in cardiovascular function: a meta-analysis." *Journal of Advancement in Medicine*, Fall 1993; Vol. 6, Number 3.

17. Chappell L.T., Stahl J.P., and Evans R. "EDTA chelation treatment for vascular disease: a meta-analysis using unpublished data." *J Adv Med*, 1994; 7(3): 131.

18. McDonagh E.W., Rudolph C.J., and Cheraskin E. "The effect of intravenous disodium ethylenediaminetetraacetic acid (EDTA) plus supportive multivitamin/trace mineral supplementation upon fasting serum calcium." *Med Hypotheses*, Aug 1983; 11(4): 431-8.

19. Schaumberg D.A., Mendes F., Balaram M., Dana M.R., Sparrow D., and Hu H. "Accumulated lead exposure and risk of age-related cataract in men." *JAMA*, 2004; 292: 2750-2754.

20. Menke, A., Muntner P., Batuman V., et al. "Blood Lead Below 0.48 µmol/L (10 µg/dL) and Mortality Among U.S. Adults." *Circulation*; 114: 1388-1394.

21. Menke, A., et al, *ibid.*

22. Gmerek D.E., et al, *ibid.*

23. Green D.J., O'Driscoll J.G., Maiorana A., Scrimgeour N.B., Weerasooriya R., Taylor R.R. "Effects of chelation with EDTA and vitamin B therapy on nitric oxide-related endothelial vasodilator function." *Clin Exp Pharmacol Physiol*, 1999 Nov; 26(11): 853-6.

24. Cranton E.M. "Introduction to the Second Edition," *A Textbook on EDTA Chelation Therapy* (Second Edition), edited by Elmer M. Cranton, Hampton Roads Publishing, Virginia, 2001, xxi-xxxviii.

25. Cranton E.M., *ibid*.

26. Carter J.P. "If EDTA Chelation Therapy Is So Good, Why Is It Not More Widely Accepted?" *A Textbook on EDTA Chelation Therapy* (Second Edition), edited by Elmer M. Cranton, Hampton Roads Publishing, Virginia, 2001: 329-342.

27. Hancke C, Flytie K. "Benefits of EDTA chelation therapy on arteriosclerosis." *J Adv Med*. 1993; 6: 161-172.

28. Lin J.L., Lin-Tan D.T., Hsu K.H., and Yu C.C. "Environmental Lead Exposure and Progression of Chronic Renal Diseases in Patients without Diabetes." *New England Journal of Medicine*, May 2003; 348: 1810-1812.

29. Lin-Tan D.T., Lin J.L., Yen T.H., Chen K.H. and Huang Y.L. "Long-term outcome of repeated lead chelation therapy in progressive non-diabetic chronic kidney diseases." *Nephrol Dial Transplant*, June 7, 2007.

Chapter 1

1. Clarke N.E., Clarke C.N., and Mosher R.E. "The "in vivo" dissolution of metastatic calcium: an approach to atherosclerosis." *Am J Med Sci*, 1955; 220: 142-149.

2. Chappell T.L. and Stahl J.P. "The correlation between EDTA chelation therapy and improvement in cardiovascular function: a meta-analysis." *Journal of Advancement in Medicine*, Fall 1993; Vol. 6, Number 3.

3. Wirebaugh S.R. and Geraets D.R. "Apparent failure of edetic acid chelation therapy for the treatment of coronary atherosclerosis." *DICP*, 1990 Jan; 24(1): 22-5.

4. Chappell T.L. and Stahl J.P., *ibid.*

5. Clarke N.E., Clarke C.N., and Mosher R.E. "Treatment of Angina Pectoris With Disodium Ethylene Diamine Tetraacetic Acid." *American Journal of the Medical Sciences*, Dec., 1956; 232: 654-666.

6. Clarke, Sr., N.E. "Atherosclerosis, occlusive vascular disease and EDTA." (Ed) *American Journal of Cardiology*, 1960; 6:233-36.

7. Clarke, Sr., N.E., Clarke, Jr., N.E., and Mosher R.E. "Treatment of occlusive vascular disease with disodium ethylenediamine tetraacetic acid (EDTA)." *American Journal of Medical Science*, 1960; 239:732-44.

8. Evers R. "Chelation of vascular atheromatous disease (experience with 3000 patients)." Am. J. Cardiol., 1960, 6: 233-236.

9. Kitchell J.R., Palmon F., Aytan N., Meltzer L.E., "The treatment of coronary artery disease with disodium EDTA, a reappraisal." *Am. J. Cardiol.*, 1963; 11:501-506.

10. Cranton E.M. "Introduction to the Second Edition," *A Textbook on EDTA Chelation Therapy* (Second Edition), edited by Elmer M. Cranton, Hampton Roads Publishing, Virginia, 2001, xxi-xxxviii.

11. Chappell T.L. and Stahl J.P., *ibid.*

12. Sincock A.M. "Life extension in the rotifer mytilina brevispina vat redunca by the application of chelating agents." *J Gerontol.*, 1975; 30: 289-293.

13. Guldager B., Jelnes R., Jorgensen S.J., et al. "EDTA treatment of intermittent claudication--a double-blind, placebo-controlled study." *Journal of Internal Medicine*, 1992; 231: 261-267.

14. Van Rij A.M., Solomon C., Packer S.G., and Hopkins W.G. "Chelation therapy for intermittent claudication. A double-blind, randomized, controlled study." *Circulation*, 1994, September; 90(3): 1194-1199.

15. Cranton E.M. and Frackelton J.P. "Negative Danish study of EDTA chelation biased." *Townsend Letter for Doctors*, July 1992; 604-605.

16. Cranton E.M. "Scientific Rationale for EDTA Chelation Therapy in

Treatment of Atherosclerosis and Diseases of Aging," *A Textbook on EDTA Chelation Therapy* (Second Edition), edited by Elmer M. Cranton, Hampton Roads Publishing, Virginia, 2001: 3-61.

17. Hancke C. and Flytie K. "Benefits of EDTA chelation therapy on arteriosclerosis." *J Adv Med*. 1993; 6: 161-172.

Chapter 2

1. Wilson, C. *Chemical Exposure and Human Health*, McFarland (Jefferson, North Carolina), 1992, 1-2.

2. Wilson, C., *ibid*.

3. Bhat R.K., et al. "Trace elements in hair and environmental exposure." *Sci Total Environ*, 1982, 22 (2): 169.

4. Batuman V., Landy E., Maesaka J.K., and Wedeen R.P. "Contribution of lead to hypertension with renal impairment." *N Engl J Med*, 1983, 309(1):17.

5. Menke, A., Muntner P., Batuman V., et al. "Blood Lead Below 0.48 µmol/L (10 µg/dL) and Mortality Among U.S. Adults." *Circulation*, 114: 1388-1394.

6. Alling A. and Nelson M. *Life Under Glass: The Inside Story of Biosphere 2*. The Biosphere Press, Oracle, Arizona, 1993.

7. Poynter J. *The Human Experiment: Two Years and Twenty Minutes Inside Biosphere 2*. Thunder's Mouth Press, New York, 2006.

8. Duncan D.E. "The Pollution Within," *National Geographic*, October, 2006; 210(4): 116-143.

9. Menke, A., Muntner P., Batuman V., et al. *ibid*.

10. Schaumberg D.A., Mendes F., Balaram M., Dana M.R., Sparrow D., and Hu H. "Accumulated lead exposure and risk of age-related cataract in men." *JAMA*, 2004; 292: 2750-2754.

11. Patterson C. and Ng A. "Natural concentrations of lead in ancient Arctic and Antarctic ice." *Geochimica et Cosmochimica Acta*, 1981; 45 (11): 2109-2121.

12. T.P. Kruck, J-G Cui, M.E. Percy and W.J. Lukiw, Molecular shuttle chelation: the use of ascorbate, desferrioxamine and Feralex-G in combination to remove nuclear bound aluminum, Cellular and Molecular *Neurobiology*, 24, (2004).

13. Hellenbrand, W., et al. "Diet and Parkinson's disease II: a possible role for the past intake of specific nutrients." *Neurology*, September 1996, 47: 644-50.

14. Johns Hopkins Medical Institutions (2007, September 12). "How Vitamin C Stops Cancer." *ScienceDaily*. Retrieved April 18, 2008, from http://www.sciencedaily.com? /releases/2007/09/070910132848.htm

15. Yeom CH, Jung GC, Song KJ (2007). "Changes of terminal cancer patients' health-related quality of life after high dose vitamin C administration". J. Korean Med. Sci. 22 (1): 7-11. PMID 17297243. Retrieved on 2007-08-03.

16. Rath MW, Pauling LC. U.S. Patent 5,278,189 Prevention and treatment of occlusive cardiovascular disease with ascorbate and substances that inhibit the binding of lipoprotein(a). USPTO. 11 Jan 1994.

17. Carr A.C. and Frei B. "Toward a new recommended dietary allowance for vitamin C based on antioxidant and health effects in humans." *American Journal of Clinical Nutrition*, June 1999, 69, 6: 1086-1107.

18. Cuvin-Aralar L. and Furness R. "Mercury and Selenium Interaction: A Review." *Ecotoxicology and Environmental Safety*, Oct 10 1990; 21: 348-364.

19. Schrauzer G.N. "Nutritional Selenium Supplements: Product Types, Quality, and Safety." *Journal of the American College of Nutrition*, 2001; 20(1): 1-4.

20. Orekhov AN, Grünwald J. "Effects of garlic on atherosclerosis." *Nutrition*, 1997 Jul-Aug; 13(7-8): 656-63.

21. Arivazhagan S., et al. "Modulatory effects of garlic and neem leaf extracts on N-methyl-N'-nitro-N-nitrosoguanidine (MNNG)-induced oxidative stress in Wistar rats," *Cell Biochem Funct*, 2000; 18 (1): 17-21.

22. Lamm, DL, and Riggs, DR. "The potential application of Allium sativum

(garlic) for the treatment of bladder cancer," *Urol Clin North Am*, 2000; 27(1): 157-162.

23. Yuriko Oi, Mika Imafuku, et al. "Garlic Supplementation Increases Testicular Testosterone and Decreases Plasma Corticosterone in Rats Fed a High Protein Diet." *Journal of Nutrition*, 2001; 131: 2150-2156.

24. Josling P. "Preventing the common cold with a garlic supplement: a double-blind, placebo-controlled survey." *Adv Ther.*, 2001 Jul-Aug; 18(4): 189-93.

25. Ide, N, and Lau, BH. "Aged garlic extract attenuates intracellular oxidative stress," Phytomedicine 6(2): 125-131, 1999.

26. Arivazhagan S., et al., *ibid.*

27. Tungland B.C. and Meyer D. "Nondigestible oligo- and polysaccharides (dietary fiber): their physiology and role in human health and food." *Comprehensive Reviews in Food Science and Food Safety*, 2002; 1: 73-92.

28. Marlett J.A. "Dietary fiber and cardiovascular disease" in *Handbook of Dietary Fiber* (edited by Cho S.S. and Dreher M.L.) Marcel Dekker, Inc, New York, 2001: 17-30.

29. Perkowski D., Wagner S., and Marcus A. "D-Ribose Improves Cardiac Indices in Patients Undergoing "Off-Pump" Coronary Arterial Revascularization," presented at Academic Surgical Congress, February, 2007.

30. Omran H., Illien S., MacCarter D., et al. "Ribose Improves Myocardial Function and Quality of Life in Congestive Heart Failure Patients." *J Mol Cell Cardiol*, 33(6): A173, 2001.

31. Cecchini M.A, Root D. A, Rachunow J. R., and Gelb P. "Chemical Exposure at the World Trade Center: Use of the Hubbard Suana Detoxification Regimen to Improve the Health Status of New York City Rescue Workers Exposed to Toxicants." *Towsend Letter for Doctors and Patients*, April 2006, 273, 58-65.

32. Walford, R. L., Mock, D., MacCallum, T., and Laseter, J. L. (1999). Physiologic changes in humans subjected to severe, selective calorie restriction for two years in Biosphere 2: Health, aging, and toxicological perspectives. *Toxicol. Sci.* 52(Suppl.), 61–65.

33. Muldoon S.B., Cauley J.A., Kuller K.H., et al. "Lifestyle and Sociodemographic Factors as Determinants of Blood Lead Levels in Elderly Women." *American Journal of Epidemiology*; 139(6): 599-608.

34. Hu H., Rabinowitz M., and Smith D. "Bone Lead as a Biological Marker in Epidemiologic Studies of Chronic Toxicity: Conceptual Paradigms" *Environmental Health Perspectives*, January, 1998; 106(1): 1-8.

35. Nash D., Magder L., et al. "Blood Lead, Blood Pressure, and Hypertension in Perimenopausal and Postmenopausal Women" *JAMA*, 2003; 289(12): 1523-1532.

35. Korrick S.A., Schwartz J., et al. "Correlates of Bone and Blood Lead Levels among Middle-aged and Elderly Women" *Am J Epidemiol*, 2002; 156: 335-343.

36. Rudolph C.J., McDonagh E.W., and Wussow D. G. "The Effect of Intravenous Disodium Ethylenediaminetetraacetic Acid (EDTA) upon Bone Density Levels." *Journal of Advancement in Medicine*, 1988; 1(2): 79-85.

Chapter 3

1. Casdorph H.R. "EDTA chelation therapy ii, efficacy in arteriosclerotic heart disease." *Journal of Holistic Medicine*, Spring/Summer 1981; (3) 1.

2. Cranton E.M. and Frackelton J.P. "Current Status of EDTA chelation therapy in occlusive arterial disease." *Journal of Holistic Medicine*, 1982; 4(1):24-33.

3. Hancke C. and Flytlie K. "Benefits of EDTA chelation therapy in arteriosclerosis: a retrospective study of 470 patients." *Journal of Advancement in Medicine*, 1993; 6(3): 161-72.

4. Born G.R., Geurkink T.L. "Improved peripheral vascular function with low dose intravenous ethylene diamine tetraacetic acid (EDTA)." *The Townsend Letter*, July, 1994: 722-726.

5. Ali M., Ale O., Fayemi A., Juco J., Grieder-Brandenburger C. "Improved myocardial perfusion in patients with advance ischemic heart disease with an integrative management program including EDTA chelation therapy." *Townsend Letter for Doctors and Patients*, January 1999.

6. Pouls M. "Oral Chelation and Nutritional Replacement Therapy for Chemical & Heavy Metal Toxicity and Cardiovascular Disease." *Townsend Letter for Doctors and Patients*, July, 1999.

7. Clarke N.E., Clarke C.N., and Mosher R.E. "The "in vivo" dissolution of metastatic calcium: an approach to atherosclerosis." *Am J Med Sci*, 1955; 220: 142-149.

8. Clarke N.E., Clarke C.N., and Mosher R.E. "Treatment of Angina Pectoris With Disodium Ethylene Diamine Tetraacetic Acid." *American Journal of the Medical Sciences*, Dec., 1956; 232: 654-666.

9. Clarke, Sr., N.E. "Atherosclerosis, occlusive vascular disease and EDTA." (Ed) *American Journal of Cardiology*, 1960; 6: 233-36.

10. Clarke, Sr., N.E., Clarke, Jr., N.E., and Mosher R.E. "Treatment of occlusive vascular disease with disodium ethylenediamine tetraacetic acid (EDTA)." *American Journal of Medical Science*, 1960; 239: 732-44.

11. Hancke C, Flytlie K. Benefits of EDTA Chelation Therapy in Arteriosclerosis: A Retrospective Study of 470 Patients. *Journal of Advancement in Medicine*. 1993; 6(3): 161-171.

12. Casdorph, R.H. "EDTA Chelation Therapy: Efficacy in Arteriosclerotic Heart Disease." *A Textbook on EDTA Chelation Therapy* (Second Edition), edited by Elmer M. Cranton, Hampton Roads Publishing, Virginia, 2001: 133-141.

13. Chappell L.T. and Stahl J.P. "The correlation between EDTA chelation therapy and improvement in cardiovascular function: a meta-analysis." *Journal of Advancement in Medicine*, Fall 1993; (6)3: 139.

14. Chappell L.T., Stahl J.P., and Evans R. "EDTA chelation treatment for vascular disease: a meta-analysis using unpublished data." *J Adv Med*, 1994; 7(3): 131.

15. Pitt B., Waters D., Brown W.V., Van Boven A.D. J., Schwartz L., et al. "Aggressive lipid-lowering therapy compared with angioplasty in stable coronary artery disease." *N Engl J Med*, 1999; 341: 70-76.

16. McDonagh E.W., Rudolph C.J., and Cheraskin E. "The effect of intravenous disodium ethylenediaminetetraacetic acid (EDTA) plus supportive multivitamin/trace mineral supplementation upon fasting serum calcium." *Med Hypotheses*, Aug 1983; 11(4): 431-8.

17. Knudtson M.L., Wyse D.G., Galbraith, P.D. "Chelation Therapy for Ischemic Heart Disease: A Randomized Controlled Trial." *JAMA*, January 23/30, 2002; 287(4) 481-486.

18. Green D.J., O'Driscoll J.G., Maiorana A., Scrimgeour N.B., Weerasooriya R., Taylor R.R. "Effects of chelation with EDTA and vitamin B therapy on nitric oxide-related endothelial vasodilator function." *Clin Exp Pharmacol Physiol*, 1999 Nov; 26(11): 853-6.

19. Vohra F. and Kratzer F.H. "Influence of various chelating agents on the availability of zinc." *J. Nutrition*; 1964, 82: 249-56.

20. Ewald P.W. *Plague Time*, Anchor Books, New York, 2002.

21. Keith A. "Regulating Information About Aspirin and the Prevention of Heart Attack." *The American Economic Review*, Vol. 85, No. 2, Papers and Proceedings of the Hundredth and Seventh Annual Meeting of the American Economic Association Washington, DC, January 6-8, 1995 (May, 1995), 96-99.

22. Keith A., *ibid*.

23. Knudtson M.L., et al., *ibid*.

Chapter 4

1. Crapper D.R., Krishman S.S., and Quittkat S. "Aluminum, neurofibrillary degeneration, and Alzheimer's disease." *Brain*, 1976; 99: 68-80.

2. Casdorph H.R. "EDTA chelation therapy ii, efficacy in brain disorders." *Journal of Holistic Medicine*, Fall/Winter, 1981; (3)2.

3. Casdorph H.R. "EDTA Chelation Therapy: Efficacy in Brain Disorders," *A*

Textbook on EDTA Chelation Therapy (Second Edition), edited by Elmer M. Cranton, Hampton Roads Publishing, Virginia, 2001.

4. Crapper D.R., Krishman, and Dalton A.J. "Aluminum distribution in Alzheimer's disease and experimental neurofibrillary degeneration." *Science*, 1973; 180: 511-13.

5. McDermott J.R., Smith A.E., Iqbal K., and Wisniewski H.W. "Brain aluminum in aging and Alzheimer's disease." *Neurology*, 1979; 29: 809-14.

6. Lanphear B.P., Hornung R., et al. "Low-Level Environmental Lead Exposure and Children's Intellectual Function: An International Pooled Analysis." *Environ Health Perspect*, 2005 July; 113(7): 894–899.

7. Casdorph H.R., 2001, *ibid.*

8. Jentsch J.D., Salameh W., and Fiske A. "Pilot Project # 1: Towards a Neurochemistry of Sociability." UCLA Center for Autism Research and Treatment, www.autism.ucla.edu/research/programs/grants1.php.

9. Johansen P.O. and Krebs T., January 12, 2007 News Item, www.maps.org/mdma

10. Fombonne E. "Is there an epidemic of autism?" *Pediatrics*. 2000; 107: 411-413.

11. Rodier P.M. and Hyman S.L. "Early environmental factors in autism." *MRDD* Res Rev. 1998; 4: 121-128.

12. Byrd R.S. "M.I.N.D. Institute Study Confirms Autism Increase," UC Davis Health System, Oct. 17, 2002, www.ucdmc.ucdavis.edu/news/mindepi_study.html.

13. Ramachandran V. S. and Oberman L.M. "Broken Mirrors: A Theory of Autism." *Scientific American*, November, 2006.

14. Wallis, C. "Does Watching TV Cause Autism?" www.time.com/time/health/article/0,8599,1548682,00.html

15. Redwood L. "Mercury and Autism: The Growing Crisis of Mercury in Children's Vaccines," *Vitamin Research News*, May 2001; (15)5.

16. Yasko A. and Gordon G. *The Puzzle of Autism*: Putting It All Together, Matrix Development Publishing, Payson, Arizona, 2006: 6-11, 18-25.

17. Ewald P.W. *Plague Time*, Anchor Books, New York, 2002.

18. Dean W. and Morgenthaler J. *Smart Drugs & Nutrients: How to Improve Your Memory and Increase Your Intelligence Using the Latest Discoveries in Neuroscience*. B&J Publications, Santa Cruz, 1991: 13-20, 109-111, 117-123.

19. Rao B., Norris J. "A Double-Blind Investigation of Hydergine in the Treatment of Cerebrovascular Insufficiency in the Elderly." *John Hopkins Medical Journal*, 1971; 130(9): 317- 323.

20. Emmenegger H., Meier-Ruge W. "The Actions of Hydergine on the Brain." *Pharmacology*, 1968, 1: 65-78.

21. Speigel R. "A Controlled Long-Term Study with Hydergine, in Healthy Elderly Volunteers." *Journal of the American Geriatrics Society*, 1983; 31(9): 549- 555.

22. Emmenegger H., *ibid*.

23. Bertoni-Freddari C., Fattoretti P., Casoli T., Spanga C., Meier-Ruge W. "Morphological Alterations of Synaptic Mitochondria During Aging." *The Effect of Hydergine Treatment in the Pharmacology of the Aging Process— Methods of Assessment and Potential Interventions*. Editors: Imre Zs-Nagy and Kenichi Kitani, New York Academy of Sciences, 1994.

24. Solomon, P.R., et al. "Ginkgo for Memory Enhancement: A Randomized Controlled Trial." *JAMA*. 2002; 288: 835-840.

25. Dean W., Morgenthaler J., and Fowkes S.W. *Smart Drugs II: The Next Generation*. Smart Publications, P.O. Box 4667, Petaluma, CA, 1993: 17-28.

Chapter 5

1. Ewald P.W. *Plague Time*, Anchor Books, New York, 2002.

2. Winslow S. G. "The effects of environmental chemicals on the immune system: A selected bibliography with abstracts." Oak Ridge, TN: Toxicology Information Response Center, Oak Ridge National Laboratory, 1981.

3. Groupe V., Engle C.G., and Gaffney P.E. "Antiviral Activity of Chelated Cobalt Against Influenza Virus." *J. Bacteriol*, 1955; 70: 623-624.

4. Wunderlich V. and Sydow G. "Disintegration of Retroviruses by Chelating Agents." Central Institute for Cancer Research, Robert-Rossle-Institute, Academy of Sciences of the German Democratic, Berlin, 1982.

5. Deucher G.P. "EDTA chelation therapy: an antioxidant strategy." *Journal of Advancement in Medicine*, 1988; 1(4): 182-190.

6. Ali M., Ali O., Fayemi A.O., et al. "Improved peripheral perfusion in patients with advanced peripheral arterial disease with an integrated management plan including EDTA chelation therapy." *J Integrative Medicine*, 1997.

7. Keller H. "Carnivora: Pharmacology and Clinical Efficacy of a Most Diverse Natural Plant Extract." *Townsend Letter for Doctors and Patients*, Nov, 2001.

8. Hammer K., et al. "Antimicrobial activity of essential oils and other plant extracts." *J Appl Microbial*, 1999, 86: 985-90.

9. Stiles J., et al. "The inhibition of Candida albicans by oregano." *J Appl Nutr*, 1995; 47: 96-102.

10. Tantatoui-Elaraki A. and Beraoud L. "Inhibition of growth and aflatoxin production in Aspergillus parasiticus by essential oils of selected plant materials." *J Environ Path Toxicol Oncol*, 1994; 13: 67-72.

11. Manohar V., et al. " Antifungal activities of origanum oil against Candida albicans." *Mol Cell Biochem*, 2001; 228: 111-17.

12. Knobloch K., et al. "Antibacterial and antifungal properties of essential oil components." *J Essent Oil Res*, 1989; 1: 119-28.

13. Knobloch K, *ibid*.

14. Baratta M.T., et al. "Chemical composition, antimicrobial and antioxidative activity of laurel, sage, rosemary, oregano and coriander essential oils." *J Essent Oil Res*, 1998; 10: 618-27.

15. Force M. et al. "Inhibition of enteric parasites by emulsified oil of oregano in vivo." *Phytother Res*, 2000; 14: 213-14.

16. Gmerek D.E., et al. "Effect of inorganic lead on rat brain mitochondrial respiration and energy production." *J Neurochem*. 1981 Mar; 36(3): 1109-13.

17. Bjorksten, J. "Possibilities and limitations of chelation as a means for life extension." *Rejuvenation*, 1980; 8:67.

18. Valenzano D.R., Terzibasi E., et al. "Resveratrol Prolongs Lifespan and Retards the Onset of Age-Related Markers in a Short-Lived Vertebrate." *Current Biology*, 2006, Feb 7; 16(3): 296-300.

19. Lagouge M, Argmann C, Gerhart-Hines Z, et al (2006). "Resveratrol improves mitochondrial function and protects against metabolic disease by activating SIRT1 and PGC-1alpha." *Cell*, 127 (6): 1109-22.

20. Baur J.A., Pearson K.J., Sinclair D.A., et al. "Resveratrol improves health and survival of mice on a high-calorie diet" *Nature*, Nov. 2006, 444, 337-342.

21. Kaeberlein, et al. "Substrate-specific activation of sirtuins by resveratrol." *J Biol Chem*, 2005, April 29; 280(17): 17038-45.

22. Cain J.C., "Miroestrol: an oestrogenic from the plant Pueraria mirifica." *Nature*, 1960; 188: 774-7.

23. Knight D.C. and Eden, J.A. "A review of the clinical effects of phytoestrogens." *Obstetrics & Gynecology*, 1996; 87(5): 897-904.

24. Kashemsanta L., Suvatabandhu K., and Airy Shaw A.K. "A new species of Pueraria (Leguminosae) from Thailand, yielding an oestrogenic principle." Kew Bull, 1952; 4: 549-51.

25. Sawatsri S., Juntayanee B., et al. "Pueruriu mirzjx promotes fibroblasts in normal breast cells and inhibits estrogen-dependent breast cancer cells." Unpublished data, 2001 (http://www.fda.gov/ohrms/dockets/dockets/95s0316/95s-0316-rpt0149-01-vol107.pdf.).

26. Lees A.J. "Selegiline hydrochloride and cognition." *Acta Neurol Scand Suppl*, 1991; 136: 91-4.

27. Knoll J. "Pharmacological basis of the therapeutic effect of (-) deprenyl in age-related neurological diseases." *Med* Res Rev (U.S.), September, 1992; 12(5): 505-24.

28. Knoll J., 1992, *ibid.*

29. Knoll J., Yen T.T., and Dallo J. "Long-lasting , true aphrodisiac effect of (-)deprenyl in sluggish old male rats." *Mod Orobl Pharmacopsychiat*, 1983; 19: 135-53.

30. Knoll J. "Extension of lifespan of rats by long-term (-)deprenyl treatment." *Mount Sinai J Med*, 1988; 55: 67-74.

31. Milgram N.W., et al. "Maintenance on L-deprenyl prolongs life in aged male rats." *Life Sciences*, 1990; 47: 415-20.

32. Knoll J., 1988, *ibid.*

33. Milgram N.W., *ibid.*

34. Maurizi C.P. "The therapeutic potential for tryptophan and melatonin: possible roles in depression, sleep, Alzheimer's disease and abnormal aging." *Med Hypotheses*, March 1990; 31(3): 233-42.

35. Diman V.M., Anisimov V.N., and Ostroumova M.N. "Increase in lifespan of rats following polypeptide pineal extract treatment." *Exp Pathology*, 1979; 17:539-45.

36. Lieberman H.R., Waldhauser F., Garfield G., et al. "Effects of melatonin on human mood and performance." *Brain* Res (Netherlands), 1984; 323(2): 201-7.

37. Dilman V.M. "Improvement of cell-mediated immunity after pineal gland extract treatment." *Vopr Oncol* (Problems of Oncology), 1977; 7: 70-72.

38. Maurizi C.P., *ibid.*

39. Pierpaoli W. The Melatonin Miracle: Nature's Age-Reversing, Disease-Fighting, Sex-Enhancing Hormone. Pocket Books, 1996.

40. Feldman H.A., Goldstein I., Hatzichristou D.G., Krane R.J., and McKinlay J.B. "Impotence and its medical and psychosocial correlates:

results of the Massachusetts Male Aging Study." *J Urol*, 1994 Jan; 151(1): 54-61.

41. Feldman H.A., Johannes C.B., Araujo A.B., et al. "Low Dehydroepiandrosterone and Ischemic Heart Disease in Middle-aged Men: Prospective Results from the Massachusetts Male Aging Study." *American Journal of Epidemiology*; 153(1): 79-89.

42. Rudman D., Feller A.G., Nagraj H.S., et al. "Effects of human growth hormone in men over 60 years old." *N Engl J Med*, 1990; 323: 1-6.

43. Liu H, Bravata DM, Olkin I, et al (2007). "Systematic review: the safety and efficacy of growth hormone in the healthy elderly." *Ann. Intern. Med.* 146 (2): 104–15.

44. Isidori A., Lo Monaco A., and Cappa M. "A study of growth hormone release in man after oral administration of amino acids." *Curr Med* Res Opinion, 1981; 7: 475.

Chapter 6

1. Russell J., Michalek J., Flechas J., et al. "Treatment of fibromyalgia syndrome with SuperMalic: A randomized, double-blind, placebo-controlled, crossover pilot study." *J Rheumatol*, 1995; 22(5): 953-7.

2. Gaby A. "Literature Review & Commentary." *Townsend Letter*, 247:28-30, February/March 2004.

3. Domingo J.L., Gomez M., Llobet J.M., Corbella J. "Influence of some dietary constituents on aluminum absorption and retention in rats." *Kidney Int*, April 1991; 39(4): 598-601.

4. Domingo J.L., Gómez M., Llobet J.M., and Corbella J. "Citric, malic and succinic acids as possible alternatives to deferoxamine in aluminum toxicity." *J Toxicol Clin Toxicol* 1988; 26(1-2): 67-79

5. Packer L., Witt E.H., and Tritschler H..J. "Alpha-lipoic acid as a biological antioxidant." *Free Radic Biol Med*, 1995; 2: 227-250.

6. Packer L. "Antioxidant properties of lipoic acid and its therapeutic effects in prevention of diabetes complications and cataracts." *Ann NYAcad Sci*, 1994 Nov 17; 738: 257-64.

7. Armstrong M. and Webb M. "The reversal of phenylarsenoxide inhibition of keto acid oxidation in mitochondrial and bacterial suspensions by lipoic acid and other disulphides." *Biochem J*, 1967; 103: 913-922.

8. Oregon State University (2008, January 17). Lipoic Acid Could Reduce Atherosclerosis, Weight Gain. ScienceDaily. Retrieved April 13, 2008, from http://www.sciencedaily.com? /releases/2008/01/080114162506.htm

9. Kagan V.E., Serbinova E.A., Forte T., Scita G., and Packer L. "Recycling of vitamin E in human low density lipoproteins." *J Lipid* Res, 1992; 33: 385-397.

10. Merin J.P., Matsuyama M., Kira T., Baba M.. and Okamoto T. "Alpha-lipoic acid blocks HIV-1 LTR-dependent expression of hygromycin resistance in THP-1 stable transformants." *Febs Letter*, 1996; 394: 9-13.

11. Han D., Tritschler J.H., Packer L. "Alpha-lipoic acid increases intracellular glutathione in human T-lymphocyte Jurkat cell line." *Biochem Biophys* Res Commun, 1995; 207: 238-264.

12. Merin J.P., *ibid*.

13. Panigrahi M., Sadguna Y., Shivakumar B.R., Kolluri S.V., Roy S., Pack L., and Ravindranath V. "Alpha-lipoic acid protects against reperfusion injury following cerebral ischenia in rats." *Brain* Res, 1996; 717: 184-188.

14. Stoll S., Hartmann H., Cohen S.A., and Muller W.E. "The potent free radical scavenger alpha-lipoic acid improves memory in aged mice: putative relationship to NMDA receptor deficits." *Pharm Biochem Behav*, 1993; 46: 799-805.

15. Loft S. and Poulsen H.E. "Cancer risk and oxidative DNA damage in man." *J Mol Med*, 1996; 74: 297-312.

16. Lykkesfeldt J., Hagen T.M., Vinarsky V., and Ames B.N. "Age-associated decline in ascorbic acid concentration, recycling, and biosynthesis in rat hepatocytes--reversal with (R)-alpha-lipoic acid supplementation." *FASEB J*, 1998; 12: 1183-1189.

17. Packer L, Tritschler HJ, Wessel K. (1997). "Neuroprotection by the metabolic antioxidant alpha-lipoic acid.". *Free Radic Biol Med*. 22(1-2): 359-78.

18. Srivastava K.C., Bordia A., and Verma S.K. "Curcumin, a major component of food spice turmeric (Curcuma longa) inhibits aggregation and alters eicosanoid metabolism in human blood platelets." Prostaglandins Leukot Essent Fatty Acids, 1995 Apr; 52(4): 223-7.

19. Moos P.J., Edes K., Mullally J.E, Fitzpatrick F.A. "Curcumin impairs tumor suppressor p53 function in colon cancer cells." *Carcinogenesis*, 2004; 25(9): 1611-7.

20. Bisht S., Feldmann G., Soni S., Ravi R., Karikari C., Maitra A., and Maitra A. "Polymeric nanoparticle encapsulated curcumin ("nanocurcumin"): a novel strategy for human cancer therapy." *J Nanobiotechnol*, 2007, April 17; 5: 3.

21. Campbell F.C. and Collett G.P. "Chemopreventive properties of curcumin." *Future Oncology*, 2005; 1(3), 405-414.

22. Chattopadhyay I., Biswas K., Bandyopadhyay U., and Banerjee R.K. "Turmeric and curcumin: biological actions and medicinal applications." *Current Science*, 2004; 87(1): 44-53.

23. Yang F., Lim G.P., Begum A.N., Ubeda O.J., et al. "Curcumin inhibits formation of amyloid beta oligomers and fibrils, binds plaques, and reduces amyloid in vivo." *J Biol Chem*, 2005 Feb 18; 280(7): 5892-901.

24. Ng T.P., Chiam P.C., Lee T., Chua H.C., Lim L., and Kua E.H. "Curry consumption and cognitive function in the elderly." *Am J Epidemiol*, 2006 Nov 1; 164(9): 898-906.

25. Ringman J.M., Frautschy S.A., Cole G.M., Masterman D.L., and Cummings J.L. "A potential role of the curry spice curcumin in Alzheimer's disease." *Current Alzheimer Research*; 2(2), 131-136.

26. Moos P.J., *ibid*.

27. Campbell F.C., *ibid*.

28. Dairam A., Limson J.L., Watkins G.M., Antunes E., and Daya S. "Curcuminoids, curcumin, and demethoxycurcumin reduce lead-induced memory deficits in male Wistar rats." *J Agric Food Chem*, 2007 Feb 7; 55(3): 1039-44.

29. Daniel S., Limson J.L., Dairam A., Watkins G.M., and Daya S. "Through metal binding, curcumin protects against lead- and cadmium-induced lipid peroxidation in rat brain homogenates and against lead-induced tissue damage in rat brain." *J Inorg Biochem*, 2004 Feb; 98(2): 266-75.

30. Aggarwal B.B., Kumar A., Aggarwal M.S., and Shishodia S. "Curcumin derived from turmeric (Curcuma longa): A spice for all seasons." *Phytopharmaceuticals in Cancer Chemoprevention*, 2005: 349-387.

31. Cha CW. "A study on the effect of garlic to the heavy metal poisoning of rat." *J Korean Med Sci*, 1987 Dec; 2(4): 213–224.

32. Dillon S.A., Burmi R.S., Lowe G.M., Billington D., and Rahman K. "Antioxidant properties of aged garlic extract: an in vitro study incorporating human low density lipoprotein." *Life Sci*, 2003 Feb 21; 72(14): 1583-94.

33. Barrie S.A., Wright J V. and Pizzorno J.D. "Effect of Garlic Oil on Platelet Aggregation, Serum Lipids and Blood Pressure in Humans." *Journal of Orthomolecular Medicine*, 1987; (2)1: 15-21.

34. Arivazhagan S., et al. "Modulatory effects of garlic and neem leaf extracts on N-methyl-N'-nitro-N-nitrosoguanidine (MNNG)-induced oxidative stress in Wistar rats." *Cell Biochem Funct*, 2000; 18(1): 17-21.

35. T.P. Kruck, J-G Cui, M.E. Percy and W.J. Lukiw, Molecular shuttle chelation: the use of ascorbate, desferrioxamine and Feralex-G in combination to remove nuclear bound aluminum, *Cellular and Molecular Neurobiology*, 24, (2004).

36. Chen S.C., Golemboski K.A., Sanders F.S., and Dietert R.R. "Persistent effect of in utero meso-2,3-dimercaptosuccinic acid (DMSA) on immune function and lead-induced immunotoxicity." *Toxicology*, 1999; 132(1): 67-79.

37. Tandon S.K., Singh S., and Jain V.K. "Efficacy of Combined Chelation in Lead Intoxication." Chemical Research in Toxicology, 1994, September/ October, (7)5, http://pubs.acs.org/cgi-bin/abstract.cgi/crtoec/1994/7/i05/f-pdf/f_tx00041a001.pdf?sessid=6006l3

38. Juresa D., Blanusa M., and Kostial K. "Simultaneous administration of sodium selenite and mercuric chloride decreases efficacy of DMSA and DMPS in mercury elimination in rats." *Toxicol Lett*, 2005; 155: 97–102.

INTERNET RESOURCES

Garry Gordon:

www.gordonresearch.com
www.longevityplus.com
www.youtube.com/watch?v=M1cM8i-C3IE

Check out Dr. Gordon's Web site for research updates on chelation therapy:
www.gordonresearch.com

David Jay Brown:

www.mavericksofthemind.com
www.sexanddrugs.info
www.animalsandearthquakes.com
www.mavericksofmedicine.com

Sara Huntley:

www.myspace.com/machineagemaya
Sara can be reached at: huntley.sara@gmail.com

Dietary Supplement Fact Sheets:

http://ods.od.nih.gov/Health_Information/Information_About_Individual_Dietary_
Supplements.aspx

Heavy Metal Screen Kits:

http://www.thewolfeclinic.com/bio-chelat/index.html
https://secure15.ozhosting.com/ionlife/_product-heavy-metal-test-kit.asp
http://www.heavymetalstest.com

A Note About Product Associations

Because of my interest in health and longevity, I've written for a number of different nutritional supplement companies over the years, and—as a science writer with a trusted reputation that I would like to maintain—I've sometimes felt like I was journalistically walking a fine line. While I would never compromise the high standards of scientific accuracy that I've set for my writing, and I would certainly never work with a company whose products I didn't think were of exceptionally high quality, I also don't want for my science writing to ever be perceived as hype or advertising. I know that my readers aren't stupid, and they can make up their own minds about whether to buy these products or to synthesize them in their own basement laboratories—so I encourage my readers to shop around and decide for themselves about oral chelation products and nutritional supplements.

—David Jay Brown

INDEX

ABOUT THE AUTHORS & ILLUSTRATOR

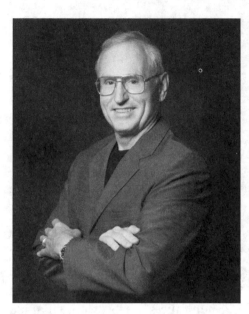

Garry Gordon, M.D., D.O., is one of the world's experts in chelation therapy, nutrition, and mineral metabolism. He is the founder and current president of the International College of Advanced Longevity Medicine (ICALM), and is one of the cofounders of the American College for Advancement in Medicine (ACAM). Dr. Gordon wrote the original protocol for the safe and effective use of EDTA oral chelation therapy, and is the author of numerous scientific papers on the subject. He is also the coauthor of the bestselling book *The Chelation Answer*.

Dr. Gordon received his Doctor of Osteopathy in 1958 from the Chicago College of Osteopathy in Illinois. In 1962 he received an honorary medical degree from the University of California, Irvine, and in 1964 he completed his Radiology Residency at Mt. Zion in San Francisco. For many years Dr. Gordon was the Medical Director of the Mineral Lab in Hayward, California, a prominent laboratory for trace mineral analysis.

Dr. Gordon is on the Board of Homeopathic Medical Examiners for Arizona, and is a Board Member of International Oxidative Medicine Association (IOMA). He is advisor to the American Board of Chelation Therapy, and was the past instructor and examiner for all chelation physicians. Dr. Gordon is responsible for Peer Review for Chelation Therapy in the State of Arizona. Dr. Gordon is currently attempting to establish standards for the proper use of oral and intravenous chelation therapy as an adjunct for treating all the major diseases. To find out more about Dr. Gordon's work visit his Web site **www.gordonresearch.com**

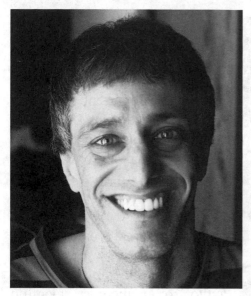

David Jay Brown is the author of four bestselling volumes of interviews with leading-edge thinkers, *Mavericks of the Mind*, *Voices from the Edge*, *Conversations on the Edge of the Apocalypse*, and *Mavericks of Medicine*. He holds a master's degree in psychobiology from New York University, worked as a neuroscience researcher in learning and memory at the University of Southern California, and was responsible for the California-based research in two of British biologist Rupert Sheldrake's books on unexplained phenomena in science: *Dogs That Know When Their Owners Are Coming Home and The Sense of Being Stared At*.

 David's work has appeared in numerous magazines, including *Scientific American Mind* and *Wired*, and he is periodically the Guest Editor of the MAPS (Multidisciplinary Association for Psychedelic Studies) *Bulletin*. David is also the author of two science fiction novels, *Brainchild* and *Virus*. To find out more about David's work visit his award-winning Web site: **www.mavericksofthemind.com**

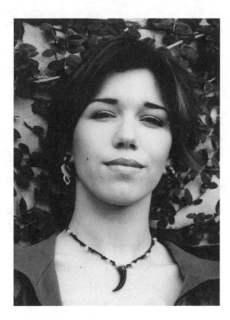

Sara Huntley is a visual artist. She is currently working on a degree in Fine Arts at the University of California, Davis, and is writing and illustrating a science fiction graphic novel. To find out more about Sara's work visit: www.myspace.com/machineagemaya Or contact Sara at: **huntley.sara@gmail.com**

PHOTO CREDITS & ILLUSTRATIONS

David Jay Brown: Photo by Deed DeBruno

Garry Gordon: Photo by Jean-Louis Husson, Feathertech.com

Sara Huntley: Photo by Jenna Sunde

All of the illustrations in this book were done by Sara Huntley.

FREE Newsletter & FREE Product Offer!

Take a moment to fill in this card and register for your free subscription to Smart Publications *Health & Wellness Update* (a $36.00 value)!   This insightful monthly newsletter provides the most blatantly honest, valuable information on nutritional medicine and health enhancement available anywhere today.

In each issue you'll receive …

*   Ground-breaking articles and interviews on today's health issues
*   Reviews of the best sources for hard-to-get nutritional supplements
*   Tips on ordering life-extending pharmaceuticals and anti-aging medicines at tremendous savings and without a prescription!

Plus, in addition to your subscription, you will also receive a coupon you can redeem for a FREE nutritional supplement from a well-known and respected nutritional supplement manufacturer.

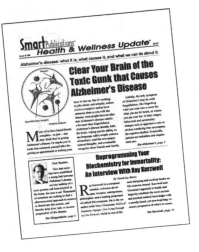

Name: _____

Company: _____

Address: _____

City/State/Zip: _____

email: _____

Title of book this page was in: <u>Detox With Oral Chelation</u>

**Simply fill out and mail this page,
and we'll rush you the latest issue…FREE!**

**Or call us, Toll Free, at 1-800-976-2783 or visit our website at
www.smart-publications.com/free to register today!**